The Treatment of Psychiatric Disorders

REVISED FOR THE *DSM-III-R*

by

William H. Reid, M.D., M.P.H.

with contributions by

George U. Balis, M.D.
James S. Wicoff, M.D.
Jerry J. Tomasovic, M.D.

BRUNNER/MAZEL, *Publishers* • New York

Library of Congress Cataloging-in-Publication Data

Reid, William H., 1945–
    The treatment of psychiatric disorders : revised for the DSM-III-R
    William H. Reid ; with contributions by George U. Balis, James S.
    Wicoff, Jerry J. Tomasovic.
        p. cm.
    Rev. ed. of: Treatment of the DSM-III psychiatric disorders.
    c1983.
    Includes bibliographies and indexes.
    ISBN 0–87630–536–2
    1. Mental illness—Treatment.   2. Diagnostic and statistical
    manual of mental disorders.   I. Reid, William H., 1945–   Treatment
    of the DSM-III psychiatric disorders.   II. Title.
    [DNLM: 1. Mental Disorders—therapy. WM 400 R359t]
    RC480.R4 1988
    616.89′1—dc19
    DNLM/DLC
    for Library of Congress   88–19468
                                                                CIP

Copyright © 1989 by William H. Reid

Published by
BRUNNER/MAZEL, INC.
19 Union Square
New York, New York 10003

MANUFACTURED IN THE UNITED STATES OF AMERICA

10   9   8   7   6   5   4   3   2   1

To Merrill T. Eaton, M.D.
to Elise
and to the memory
of Ann Alhadeff

Contents

List of Tables

Acknowledgments

R. James Willis ably organized our clinical office to accommodate this project, juggling schedules and tasks as needed. Vicki Spencer typed and retyped most of the manuscript, and was available with her word processor seven days a week. Medical student David Genecov assisted in library research. Several colleagues read and corrected early drafts.

All of these are acknowledged with thanks, but none more than my wife, Elise, who tolerated my multiple personalities of physician, medical director, writer, editor and husband—each with attendant moods and foibles—up to 18 hours a day, week in and week out, for far too long.

Contributors

William H. Reid, M.D., M.P.H., Medical Director, Colonial Hills Hospital; Clinical Professor of Psychiatry, University of Texas Health Science Center, San Antonio, Texas.

George U. Balis, M.D., Professor of Psychiatry, University of Maryland School of Medicine, Baltimore, Maryland.

James S. Wicoff, M.D., Clinical Psychiatry Faculty, Department of Psychiatry, University of Texas Health Science Center; Child and Adolescent Unit Medical Chief, Colonial Hills Hospital, San Antonio, Texas.

Jerry J. Tomasovic, M.D., Clinical Associate Professor of Pediatrics, Child Neurology Section, University of Texas Health Science Center, San Antonio, Texas.

Introduction to the Revised Edition

When I was asked to prepare a revision of *Treatment of the DSM-III Psychiatric Disorders*, in which the therapeutic modalities would be updated and keyed to the *DSM-III-R*, I asked the same questions with which the earlier volume was begun: Is there a need for this book? What is the appropriate format?

The broad readership of the first book implies a clear need. A general acceptance of its format (with notable exceptions which have been addressed herein) seems to mean that we were on the right track.

The primary author and other contributors assume that the reader is familiar with psychiatric evaluation and with the diagnostic format of *DSM-III-R*. He or she should be pursuing treatment approaches with clear working diagnoses in mind before picking up this book. The text recommends, describes, and briefly expands upon treatment modalities; however, *we make no attempt to present a complete discussion of specific treatment modalities.* This book is a guide, not a reference text.

Several thousand references, most published after 1983, were consulted. Almost 1,000 are listed within these pages. It is strongly recommended that the clinician consult these and other standard sources for more detailed information.

Virtually all standard treatment modalities, and a number of esoteric ones, have been included. Some experimental or unproved therapies are mentioned; every effort has been made to identify them as such.

It is important for the reader to note that this volume takes the extremely simplistic stance that the disorder to be treated has been accurately diagnosed according to *DSM-III-R* criteria, and that the *DSM-III-R* criteria are clinically adequate. As every clinician knows, initial diagnostic impressions are not cast in stone. A patient's response to a particular treatment may confirm, refute, or add to one's diagnosis.

In addition, it is vital that the clinician (or other reader of this book) be aware that the *DSM-III-R* is not the last or only word in our understanding of mental disorders. Diagnosis and treatment are dynamic and multifaceted, and not nearly so concrete as a lay reader might assume.

There is no real substitute for psychiatric training and experience in the treatment of most psychiatric disorders. Accordingly, although this book may be useful for general physicians or certain nonmedical mental health clinicians, it is not intended to take the place of consultation from or referral to a psychiatrist, nor is it intended for use by superficially trained counselors. The treatment techniques are for the most part intended for clinical environments, and not lay counseling centers or self-help settings.

There is particular danger of misunderstanding diagnostic and treatment concepts in legal settings. It should be made clear from the outset that this book, like the *DSM-III-R*, should not be used in the legal arena without psychiatric consultation.

Finally, there are many ways to approach the writing of a book such as this. One is to have each section or subsection written by a different expert. Although this works well for large, comprehensive texts, the variability and loss of continuity that one finds in edited texts was considered unacceptable for our purposes. I hope that readers and reviewers will agree.

William H. Reid, M.D., M.P.H.
San Antonio, TX

Prologue: The Treatment of Psychiatric Disorders

Before we present the disorders and their treatments, it is appropriate that a number of concepts that override specific treatments, and that appear again and again in the care of psychiatric patients, be discussed.

Hospitalization
Whether or not to hospitalize the patient is often a critical treatment decision. The various purposes of hospitalization include protection or monitoring of the patient, protection of others in the environment, increasing the effectiveness or efficiency of treatment, and providing certain kinds of care not available outside the hospital. Modern medical practice has given rise to some other, less acceptable reasons for hospitalization as well: convenience for the physician, convenience for the family, and increased reimbursement from third-party payers.

This creates something of a paradox. We are taught in medical training, and the public is convinced through the news media, that unnecessary hospitalization produces a tremendous drain upon our financial resources. Health care costs, which appear to be borne by insurers, employers, and governments, are in the last analysis actually carried by the taxpayer and employee. Waste and increased costs of health care are universally decried.

On the other hand, the providing of health care and its accoutrements is big business. Those whose incomes depend upon hospitalized patients, prescribed medications, or expensive procedures encourage the doctor or other clinician to use them. Thus in the private sector, one sometimes finds incentives to hospitalize which are not related to the patient's clinical needs. In the public sector (and in that portion of the private sector that is driven by cost control mechanisms such as capitation), one finds discouragements for hospitalization, many of which are not related to clinical need either.

The decision to hospitalize should be made by the *physician*, and not by administrative, political, marketing, or profit motives. The questions to ask are fairly simple. Is hospitalization the best way to treat my patient? If cost is a factor, pro or con, can cost be appropriately weighed in the clinical balance (e.g., would money saved by treatment on an outpatient basis be justified by the treatment received?)? Am I being honest with the patient and the payer in my explanation of the clinical benefits of hospital care?

The type of hospital or clinical service one uses is perhaps just as important as the decision whether or not to hospitalize. The usefulness of certain kinds of inpatient milieux in various disorders is discussed at various points in this book.

One finds considerable pressure from payers to make hospitalization as brief as possible. Most psychiatric training stresses an acute-care setting followed by outpatient or partial hospital management. For many patients, this is best. It would be a serious mistake, however, to ignore the dangers of premature discharge and the benefits of lengthy hospitalization for some patients. It has long been known that a common source of relapse is incomplete inpatient treatment, coupled with slipshod transition to the outpatient environment.

Partial Hospitalization
Partial hospital settings are very effective for some patients. It is important that the clinician seek partial hospitalization as an active, dynamic treatment setting in which the patient is clearly moving from need for the institution toward ability to function independently. This requires specialized settings, staff, and therapeutic concepts.

Unfortunately, two problems are eroding public (and payer) confidence in the partial hospitalization concept, and threaten loss of funding for these programs. One is that the common partial hospital "program" is really a halfway house for chronically ill patients. Although such settings may provide sheltered living, they must be differentiated from programs whose goal is actual patient growth.

The second problem is the program that has been specifically created to increase funding to a hospital or clinical entity. It is a fact of life that as reimbursement for some forms of treatment, such as inpatient care, becomes scarce, programs such as partial hospitalization may be established more for financial than for therapeutic reasons.

Other Treatment Settings
There are a number of treatment settings that psychiatrists use every day, but may not recognize as such. The importance of paying attention to, and sometimes guiding, the home, school, or work environment has been particularly brought out in Dr. Wicoff's section. One should always remember that the patient spends far more time with his family, his work, or his schooling than he does with any therapist. Understanding their usefulness, and sometimes their pitfalls, is critical to optimal care.

Kinds of Treaters
As mentioned in the introduction, this book is written primarily for the psychiatrist or psychiatric subspecialist. Psychiatrists in training and general physicians or medical students learning about the specialty are included in this group.

Psychiatry realizes, perhaps more than any other specialty, the importance of integrating the biological, psychological, and social facets of the patient's disorder and his life. This leads to the many advantages of multidisciplinary treatment teams, and to the psychiatrist's acceptance of the fact that some aspects of care may best be carried out by nonphysicians. The clinical psychologist or social worker trained in psychotherapy, for example, can provide treatment for many kinds of patients. Some highly specialized nonphysicians offer modalities, such as biofeedback or covert sensitization, which are often not available in the psychiatrist's office.

All of the nonmedical professionals to whom this book refers should, like psychiatrists and other physicians, be aware of the limits of their expertise and ability to help particular patients. The availability of consultants in other fields, and the willingness to use them, is very important. One's familiarity with his or her consultants should include not only knowledge of their training and credentials, but also of clinical reputation, rapport with patients, and professional ethics.

Many other people, some professional and some not, come into the treatment environment. All deserve the clinician's cooperation, in the patient's interest and in the interest of simple courtesy. Issues of privacy and confidentiality should be considered in all communications with therapists, counselors, clergy, friends, and family.

Patients and Clients

The word "patient" is used throughout this book to describe those people who have come to us for help or who are being treated. The word "client" is popular in some psychotherapeutic and counseling environments. One advantage of "client" is that it connotes a partnership between the clinician and the person being treated, providing the latter with a certain respect and responsibility for his life and care. On the other hand, it is this author's belief that the "doctor-patient" relationship has many advantages in most therapeutic and treatment settings. One's status as "patient" should not be used to infantilize or demean him or her; however, the expectations (some of which are legal ones) of "doctor" and "patient" have great value to patient care.

Diagnostic Accuracy in Treatment

Diagnosis is a cornerstone of effective treatment. The practice of psychiatry and psychotherapy is not an informal, "let's-try-this-and-see-if-it-works" endeavor. Our treatment modalities are not so broadly successful that they can be applied to anyone who happens to have particular symptoms.

The other side of the same coin is the recent effort to reduce diagnostic methods to such pseudoscientific levels that diagnoses can be made, literally, by computer. While there can be no doubt that the *reliability* of diagnosis can be improved with the use of highly standardized checklists and the like, the result is only a statistical one, and often lacks *validity*. One can program the computer to add two and two and come up with five time after time. Nevertheless, the result will not be valid.

Diagnosis must blend the best scientific methods with clinical experience, to lead to treatment decisions most likely to help the patient. If one's diagnosis is wrong, then the treatment is likely to be ineffective, partially effective at best, or even harmful. It is not so simple as merely trying a treatment to see if it works, then abandoning it after a few hours or days. Many of the treatments used in psychiatry—biological as well as psychotherapeutic ones—are complex, easy to apply incorrectly, and/or take considerable time to evaluate.

Psychiatric disorders rarely exist in a vacuum. This is true in other medical specialties as well; the pediatrician knows that while treating strep throat, he or she must consider the possibilities of kidney damage, rheumatic heart disease, and medication side effects and interactions. Psychiatric disorders seem often to be even more confusing, and present more often in combination, than many other illnesses.

It is thus extremely important that the reader not become enamored with the apparently "cookbook" style with which this book follows the DSM-III-R diagnoses. There are warnings and suggestions throughout the book regarding this; however, it bears mention here as well. The patient's overt symptoms and signs are often part of an Axis I disorder. All of this is laid over the patient's personality, which may or may not imply an Axis II diagnosis. Axis III diagnoses may be critical to one's understanding of the patient. Finally, the Axis IV and Axis V considerations of the *Diagnostic and Statistical Manual of Mental Disorders* should always be considered as one attempts to plan the best overall treatment for the individual patient.

Continua in Diagnosis and Treatment

The concept of related symptoms and disorders, and that of symptoms being laid over personality styles, organic illness, sociocultural issues, and so forth, sometimes make one think of some disorders as on a "continuum" of diagnoses. For example, at one time it was thought that neurotic illnesses, personality disorders, and psychotic illnesses merely represented differences in degree of the same basic emotional problems.

With some notable exceptions, the concept of diagnostic continua has more problems than advantages for the person who is learning about psychiatric diagnosis and treatment. It is better to understand separately, for example, the characteristics and treatment of schizophrenic patients, schizoid patients, "borderline" patients with brief psychotic episodes, and severely anxious patients whose symptoms reach psychotic proportions. When exceptions to this general rule exist, they will be mentioned in the text.

Pessimism vs. Realism in Treatment

Although, taken as a group, psychiatric disorders have about the same rate of cure or amelioration of discomfort as those found in other medical specialties, they are often viewed more pessimistically. The vast majority of patients with psychiatric disorders *are* treatable, given appropriate diagnosis and resources for treatment. It is important to recall that the relief of pain, mental or physical, with or without a "cure," is often the physician's highest calling.

Treating the "Myth of Mental Illness"

Psychiatry is perhaps the only clinical field in which aberrant behavior or emotions alone can warrant a "diagnosis" and "treatment." Although this author acknowledges the importance of sociocultural factors in determining whether a particular feeling or behavior (or even an hallucination) is or is not normal, mental illness is not a "myth." The longer a clinician works with patients; sees the interaction of biological, psychological and social factors in their pain; and sees the patterns of disturbance which appear over and over; the more he or she becomes convinced that mental disorders deserve consideration beyond labels of maladaptation or "problems in living."

On the other hand, the clinician who has the social (and perhaps legal) authority to diagnose and treat such disorders must take this responsibility very seriously. The international literature is rife with situations in which social or political behavior is confused with illness. The issue of using psychiatry to control behavior is one that deserves more space than is available in this book; however, one should be particularly careful when treating children, adolescents, the elderly, and people whose behavior is deemed "antisocial."

The Treatment of Psychiatric Disorders

REVISED FOR THE *DSM-III-R*

Section I:
Disorders Usually
First Evident in Infancy,
Childhood, or Adolescence

by

James S. Wicoff, M.D.

Several factors must be taken into account that are somewhat limited in treating children and adolescents and may call for a different perspective from that used in treating adults. First of all, the rapidly changing physical and psychological makeup of the child often influences the choice of treatment for a particular psychopathology. Second, while chemical research has progressed a great deal in general psychiatry and application to adults, research about and application to children still lag quite far behind. This is due, in part, to regulations governing experimentation with medications in children, as well as to the above-mentioned rapidly changing nature of the child's physiology. Psychotropic intervention, therefore, is not as well documented in either clinical trials or long-term follow-up studies. The third factor that is unique to treating children and adolescents is the routine inclusion of family members in the treatment process. Family therapy and/or education is generally crucial to any therapeutic approach used with children and adolescents.

DRUG TREATMENT IN CHILDREN

Although the body of knowledge regarding psychotropic medications has expanded tremendously over the last 30 years, the use of these medications in children has not been nearly as well studied. Many factors contribute to this, including the rarity in children of some disorders such as manic-depressive illness and schizophrenia and parents' resistance to the use of psychotropic medicines. Studies of the medication effects on control groups are difficult to find.

Nevertheless, there is growing use of the full range of psychotropic medications in child and adolescent psychiatry. Clinicians prescribing for this age group should be well aware of the developmental variations, both physical and psychological, seen in children and adolescents and the effects these have on the presentation of their disorders. There should also be careful consideration of the family's influence on the placebo effects of the medication. Children are strongly influenced by the introduction of the medication and family support for their taking it.

Education of both the child and the family about the medication and what it can and cannot accomplish is crucial to obtaining optimal effects of the drug. Questions about short- and long-term side effects and possible predisposition to substance abuse in adolescents should be answered straightforwardly and the drug should not be started until the family is in support of its use. During the first few weeks of treatment the family should be encouraged to call whenever they have questions. The physician should be readily available and able to answer questions regarding side effects, interactions with other medications, and other concerns of either parent or child.

Whenever possible, a single daily dose should be given to avoid having the child leave class to take medication. Initiation of medications is generally best done at doses below therapeutic amounts, to avoid initial side effects and related rejection of the drug. The dose should

be increased systematically once or twice a week until positive therapeutic effects are noted, or unacceptable side effects are experienced.

Assessment of efficacy must often be done through communication
with the school. This is the one place where the child experiences a
consistent and repetitive level of task orientation, peer interaction, and
academic stress. Teachers, however, may have previously fixed opinions
about the use of medications in children. One should use structured
rating methods such as questionnaires which allow for objective monitoring of the child's progress.

The preschool child who is taking medication often develops behavioral toxicity. This usually takes the form of either increased or
decreased activity, loss of appetite, or general irritability. Symptoms
such as these should lead the clinician to reduce the dosage or eliminate
the medicine for several days, then try restarting at a lower dose.

Long-term side effects are often asked about by parents who have
seen reports in popular magazines or on television. Although systematic
studies of most drugs are at best inconsistent, we can say that side
effects such as extrapyramidal signs and tardive-dyskinesia-like syndromes are not seen as often in adolescents as they are in adults, and
that the frequency generally decreases with the age of the child. This
is also true for impaired liver functioning, jaundice, and bone marrow
damage. Stunting of growth by stimulants is also brought up quite
often. Follow-up studies to the original paper that postulated growth
retardation have indicated that stimulants may reduce weight gain, but
that height is not affected (Gross, 1976; McNutt et al., 1976; Quinn &
Rapoport, 1975). Side effects with methylphenidate generally do not
occur if the dose remains around 0.3 mg/kg/day. When the dose is
increased to 1.0 mg/kg/day, over 50% of children have some side
effect (worsening of behavior, weight loss, or general irritability).

One should consider discontinuing stimulants for one to two weeks
in the fall after the first six weeks of school and in the spring a few
weeks before or after spring break. This allows determination of continuing necessity of the drug. The teacher should be informed of the
trial period in order to be more observant and tolerant of the child's
behavior during this time. Should the behavior be intolerable after only
a few days, medication can easily be restarted.

Two medications that are used quite often by pediatricians and
should be considered in behavior control are chloral hydrate and diphenhydramine. Chloral hydrate can be prescribed in doses of 25–50
mg/kg/day, divided into two or three doses for sedative and/or hypnotic effects, in emergency situations or treatment of insomnia. Di-

phenhydramine is usually given in much smaller doses for an anti-histaminic, but can be used in dosages from 3–26 mg/kg/day for behavioral control. This is particularly effective in children with hyperactivity who are not responsive to other medication approaches.

Lithium carbonate is being used more and more in childhood disorders that are either diagnosed as bipolar illness or resemble it in terms of severe mood swings. Lithium has not been found to be effective in the Attention Deficit-Hyperactive Disorder child. Prescribing lithium for children should be limited to psychiatrists with experience with both children and the medication, and good laboratory evaluation should be available. Hospitalization for establishment of dose ranges is often needed.

Therapies using megavitamins, "natural" diets, sugar restrictions, or hypoallergenic diets have been suggested for several disorders. To this point, none has proved consistently effective.

Medication usage in children and adolescents is often warranted for the more severe behavioral disorders and, in particular, for hyperactivity. Medicine by itself, however, is never the sole treatment for these children and should be prescribed in conjunction with individual, family, group, or educational therapies.

ADULT DISORDERS IN CHILDREN

Several adult diagnoses found in *DSM-III-R* (American Psychiatric Association, 1987) will occasionally be applied to the child or adolescent. Schizophrenia is rarely found in early childhood, but when it does occur it is severely disruptive to the entire family. Treatment often involves hospitalization, the use of neuroleptics, and long-term therapy. Family therapy is essential to evaluate the psychopathology of the environment, to determine changes that may be necessary in the child's placement, or to ameliorate aberrant communication or disturbance in the parents.

The same can be said of bipolar illness in children. This diagnosis should be considered more often when there is a clear family history of bipolar illness. Lithium carbonate can be valuable in the treatment of these children.

Major Affective Disorder, Dysthymic Disorder, and the Personality Disorders are also diagnosable in children and adolescents, but are rare compared to most others that we diagnose.

Chapter 1

Developmental Disorders (Axis II)

The use of the term "Developmental Disorders" may be misleading to the parent or lay individual. The concept of a developmental disorder may indicate to them that their child will "grow out" of the problem. While this may be true at times, these disorders are generally chronic in nature and persist in some form into adult life. The use of ongoing evaluative procedures and new diagnostic workups every 18 months to 3 years is helpful not only in evaluating one's therapeutic interventions, but also in being able to answer family members' questions with regard to possible prognosis.

1A: MENTAL RETARDATION
There are no changes in the diagnosis of Mental Retardation from what is described in *DSM-III*. *DSM-III-R* indicates that the essential features of this disorder are:

> (1) Significantly subaverage general intellectual functioning accompanied by (2) significant deficits or impairment in adaptive functioning, with (3) onset before the age of 18. The diagnosis is made regardless of whether or not there is a co-existing physical or other mental disorder. (p. 28)

There have been numerous studies demonstrating the high frequency of psychiatric disorders in the mentally retarded. Emphasis has been placed on the much-increased prevalence (47% by some studies) of these disorders in the severely retarded. Childhood psychosis, severe Stereotypy/Habit Disorder, Pica, Behavioral Disorders, and isolated habits all appear to be more common than in normal intelligence children. The psychiatrist, therefore, must be prepared to deal therapeutically with a wide range of emotional and behavioral disturbances, and yet a diminished ability of the individual to deal verbally or behaviorally with stress. Assessment and treatment, however, should start with the same techniques one uses with the normal intellect child and then be modified according to the patient's particular limitations. The following guidelines help define treatment choices:

317.00   Mild Mental Retardation

This category of individuals comprises approximately 85% (American Psychiatric Association, 1987, p. 32) and, therefore, the largest group of mentally retarded individuals. Advances in the understanding and treatment of mental retardation have led to much higher goals for this group which used to be termed "educable." Parents can now be told that these children, with good intervention and programming, can generally live successfully in the community as adults either "independently or in supervised apartments or group homes" (American Psychiatric Association, 1987, p. 32). The key to achieving this goal for the mildly retarded is a team approach with careful testing to properly place the child in a situation that he or she can handle. Early diagnosis helps this a great deal, and careful explanation to the parents of their child's academic and social limitations and potentials will help the parents not only adjust their expectations, but also be realistic advocates for their child in school and social environments. Avoiding excessive exposure to failure through unrealistic parental or environmental expectations can help the individual child or adolescent immensely (Carr, 1980).

When psychiatric disturbances do occur in the mildly retarded, they are generally handled with more emphasis on family therapy and behavior modification, but individual psychotherapy and use of medication are also quite important. Individual therapy is often in the form of play therapy, to circumvent the need for frequent verbal responses by the individual and also as a more developmentally appropriate technique. Any drug therapy should be monitored closely, because of the patient's difficulty at times verbalizing side effects and the tendency of those around the child toward complacency in letting the drug become the sole therapeutic agent. Here again, family education is very important, as the parents will often be the ones to note side effects in their children that others in the environment may not perceive.

Behavioral modification is a cornerstone for the treatment of many psychiatric disturbances in the mildly retarded, such as Conduct Disorders and Stereotypy/Habit Disorders (Yule & Carr, 1980). Parents who are willing and able to learn the tenets of behavioral modification often become quite creative behavioral therapists and are able to handle many of the day-to-day problems that arise with their children without the need for professional help.

318.00 Moderate Mental Retardation

This group of individuals (formerly referred to as "trainable") is more severely limited verbally. Thus, treatment interventions shift toward the increased use of behavioral interventions and environmental support systems. Psychopathology is often more prominent and requires institutionalization more often than in the mildly retarded.

Supportive therapy with parents in dealing with their despair and sense of helplessness is very important. Community agencies can often be beneficial in alleviating the financial and emotional stresses that these families undergo. Respite programs in local hospitals or mutual support groups among parents often give families a needed rest from taking care of their handicapped child. This in turn allows them to give energies to their marriages and/or their nonhandicapped children, helping avoid the buildup of anger and resentment that often occurs when a severely handicapped child is in the home.

318.10 Severe Mental Retardation

This group of individuals, a small minority of the people with Mental Retardation, need a much more extensive network of support in the community and at home. They will need constant supervision even as adults, but can often adapt well to life in the community. Almost half of these individuals will at some time develop a psychiatric disorder and be in need of a mental health specialist. Drug therapy and behavior modification are the most frequently used interventions with these disorders, whether it be childhood psychosis or Attention-Deficit Hyperactivity Disorder. The drugs used are no different than those used to treat the same psychiatric disturbances in the regular population. Proper dosages, however, seem to be quite difficult to maintain. The mentally retarded child often has an initial reduction of symptoms, but then seems to need larger doses of medicine than his or her average-intellect counterpart (Lipton et al., 1977). There appears to be a very narrow range of efficacy for the major tranquilizers. Thioridazine and haloperidol have become the two most commonly used medications. Thioridazine has been particularly helpful in reducing stereotypy and tics. Haloperidol has been useful in treating psychosis, both because of its potency and its ease of administration in colorless drops, or intramuscularly. Minor tranquilizers and antidepressants are generally not indicated in retarded children. Exceptions to this statement would be clearcut evidence of affective illness or use of imipramine for nocturnal enuresis. Stimulant medications are not as effective for the most part in controlling hyperactivity as one sees in their use in normal children. There is also an increased risk of stereotyped behavior when stimulants are used in the severely retarded patient.

In all cases, a behavior modification program is essential as an adjunct to any drug therapy. The use of operant conditioning techniques can often reduce the need for medications. These techniques involve careful analysis of the retarded child's behavior, in both its antecedents and its consequences. The child's particular intellectual level will dictate whether more sophisticated systems such as the use of tokens can be employed. Individual therapy can be used at a very basic play therapy level. Family education becomes crucial in teaching the families to adapt to particular limitations of the individual and also to continue a home treatment program after any kind of institutionalization.

318.20   Profound Mental Retardation
These individuals comprise approximately 1%–2% of those with Mental Retardation and are generally institutionalized. They need a great deal of structure in their environment and if they develop psychiatric disorders, they often need institutionalization in a facility trained to deal with the "dually diagnosed" mentally retarded. Therapeutic interventions center around medications to control violent physical outbursts or self-destructive habits. Behavior modification, here again, is a cornerstone of working with these individuals and someone with higher level training in this area is generally needed to set up a program to deal with the sometimes complex behavioral problems. These may range anywhere from encopresis and enuresis to psychotic outbursts.

319.00   Unspecified Mental Retardation
This category is used for infants and those who are untestable but presumed to be mentally retarded. The above mentioned tenets of therapeutic intervention still apply in this category. Diagnostic evaluations (neurological, genetic, biochemical) will often dictate the direction in which therapeutic intervention proceeds.

Drug Therapy in Mental Retardation
The use of medications in the mentally retarded is often more complex than when treating a child or adolescent of normal intellectual abilities. The lack of verbal feedback regarding the child's experience of side effects or understanding of the purpose of the medication often handicaps the physician in evaluating his or her treatment. In addition, it has been demonstrated that the mentally retarded often have unusual responses to medications, or very small therapeutic windows. Complicating matters even further is the increased incidence of neurological problems, such as epilepsy. Anticonvulsant therapy needs to be monitored quite closely with blood levels for possible toxicity and/or side effects, as well as interactions with psychotropics such as phenothiazines which can change the seizure threshold. The high doses of neuroleptics often needed for reduction of self-destructive behavior in the mentally retarded make these individuals at increased risk for long-term side effects, such as tardive dyskinesia, blood dyscrasias, and liver disorders. Regular blood counts and chemical profiles followed by complete physical checkups by a physician are all very important in the treatment. The prescribing physician should also be quite cautious about lapsing into the complacency of "medication only" intervention. This can lead to higher and higher doses of neuroleptics when behavioral interventions or decreased dosage could possibly reduce or eliminate the need for medications.

Perhaps the most disturbing psychiatric syndrome that develops in the retarded is severe self-destructive behavior such as head-banging, biting of oneself, or other self-mutilation. Newer medication approaches to these symptoms are currently revolving around the use of lithium, propanolol, or carbamazepine. All of these medications are used in dosages that can either be increased to the maximum recommended blood levels, as in the case of Tegretol and lithium, or until side effects or improvement is seen in the case of propanolol. Psychotic symptoms in the individual should point toward a first-line use of major tranquilizers. Thioridazine and haloperidol are chosen medications by many physicians dealing with the retarded, but this is often because of their availability in a palatable liquid form. Other major tranquilizers can be equally effective.

1B: PERVASIVE DEVELOPMENTAL DISORDERS
This diagnostic category in *DSM-III-R* is being used to pull together a number of different early childhood disorders characterized by "qualitative impairment in the development of reciprocal social interaction,

in the development of verbal and nonverbal communication skills, and in imaginative activity" (p. 33). Old diagnostic terms such as atypical development, symbiotic psychosis, childhood psychosis, childhood schizophrenia, and autism will all now be subsumed under Pervasive Developmental Disorders. Careful attention should be paid to the introductory pages in the *DSM–III–R* which help one to understand the thinking behind this diagnostic category and the complications involved in differential diagnosis and prediction of future adaptation and general prognosis.

299.00   Autistic Disorder
Please note the revised criteria for diagnosis of this disorder. The old diagnosis of Childhood Onset Pervasive Developmental Disorder is now included under autism and the age of onset criterion has been dropped because of the inability of researchers to validate this as a predictable criterion.

Treatment of autistic disorders over the past 30 years has varied greatly as a result of conflicting theories regarding etiology, diagnosis, and prognosis. Experimentation with physiological interventions such as LSD, ECT, and numerous other medications reflects the confusion that has existed. Currently, the use of fenfluramine (a drug that reduces serotonin levels) is being considered. Thus far, the results seem to be short-term and difficult to replicate, but have been occasionally encouraging. The overall treatment of autism is summarized quite well by Rutter and Hersov in *Child and Adolescent Psychiatry* (1985).

Treatment is centered around the long-term benefits of an intensive, behaviorally oriented treatment program. Emphasis is placed on the use of techniques appropriate to the level and pattern of the children's cognitive handicaps. A child's IQ level is deemed important in terms of possible goals. An IQ below 50 generally indicates an inability, no matter what the program, to attain any kind of useful skill in reading, writing, and arithmetic. Following are the goals, strategies, and principles of treatment summarized by Rutter (1985):

The Fostering of Normal Development. This involves attending to the cognition, language, and socialization areas of development and finding ways to reduce or circumvent the effects of autism in these areas. Language development and socialization skills are concentrated on through behavioral techniques and teaching parents alternative methods of being directly and, sometimes intrusively, involved in their child's development in these areas.

The Promotion of Autistic Children Learning More Generally.
Teaching the autistic child involves breaking down learning tasks into
very small steps with high rates of success. Autistic children tend to
retreat into stereotypys when they face failure.

The Reduction of Rigidity in Stereotypy. This problem is best
approached with a very stimulated environment that goes about ac-
complishing changes through very small steps, each of which by itself
does not upset the child as it does not indicate any noticeable change
in their environment. Stereotypies can be reduced and/or modified to
more acceptable expressions through this technique.

The Elimination of Nonspecific Maladaptive Behaviors. These
involve behaviors such as tantrums, aggression, bedwetting, and encopresis. The behavioral approaches used for these problems are also
used in the case of autism with some minor modifications.

The Alleviation of Family Distress. This may be the most important component of the treatment in that family understanding of
the child's problems and needs helps create a more supportive environment both from the parents and from siblings. Several sessions
should be spent with the family going over diagnostic studies and
talking about the future.

Drug intervention with the autistic child should be for the specific
type of problem manifested. This is difficult, however, when one speaks
of symptoms such as attention deficit and stereotypy/habits that require
knowledge of not only the autistic symptomatology, but also comparative
developmental levels. There is some indication that attention deficit in
the autistic child, for instance, does not respond to normal levels of
stimulant medication. One must weigh, therefore, the benefits and risks
of high doses of medications like methylphenidate when trying to help
the autistic child to have a longer attention span in an academic or
home setting. In general, stimulants are contraindicated as a treatment
of hyperactivity because they tend to increase stereotypy/habit disorders.

Self-mutilation is the symptom that causes the most concern in the
autistic child's environment. Use of protective devices (helmets, gloves,
etc.), drug intervention, and behavioral modification can generally reduce
or eliminate the self-mutilating behavior. Phenothiazines are considered
safer than the butyrophenones, although the latter can be more powerful.

299.80   Pervasive Developmental Disorder Not Otherwise Specified

This category of individuals is considered a diagnostic dilemma, but is used for children who have enough qualitative impairments in development that they deserve a Pervasive Developmental Disorder diagnosis. The long-term outcome for these children is much more variable; continual evaluation and the therapeutic interventions outlined above are essential to allowing the highest level of potential for the individual.

1C: SPECIFIC DEVELOPMENTAL DISORDERS

These disorders are much more specific for a certain type of developmental problem such as academic, language, speech, or motor skills than the foregoing.

ACADEMIC SKILLS DISORDERS

315.10   Developmental Arithmetic Disorder
315.80   Developmental Expressive Writing Disorder
315.00   Developmental Reading Disorder

LANGUAGE AND SPEECH DISORDERS

315.39   Developmental Articulation Disorder
315.31   Developmental Expressive Language Disorder
315.31   Developmental Receptive Language Disorder

MOTOR SKILLS DISORDER

315.40   Developmental Coordination Disorder
315.90   Specific Developmental Disorder Not Otherwise Specified (NOS)

Therapeutic intervention for these disorders is generally not handled by the mental health professional. Education specialists or perhaps neurologists are the first people to see these children. The psychiatrist or mental health professional is often brought in when associated psychiatric disturbances are suspected. Psychiatric presentation most commonly takes the form of Conduct Disorders. The child with a

Chapter 10

Delirium and Dementia

10A: DELIRIUM

Most of the causes of Organic Mental Disorders listed in Table 1 may result in delirium, acting alone or in combination with several other factors (multifactorial etiology). Its most common etiology involves drugs (Table 2). Various metabolic disorders, infectious diseases, endocrinopathies, systemic disorders, and primary CNS disorders (including infections, head trauma, postictal syndromes, neoplasms, and cerebrovascular disorders) are also relatively common (Table 1).

General Therapeutic Principles

The treatment and management of the delirious patient are generally based upon the following therapeutic principles:

1. Identify and treat the causative factor(s) of the underlying primary disorder;
2. Understand the pathogenic mechanisms of the disease process that led to the development of the delirium;
3. Recognize emergency situations for early treatment intervention (e.g., hypoxia, hypoglycemia) in order to prevent the possibility of irreversible brain damage (e.g., dementia) or death.
4. Recognize and treat those psychiatric symptoms that must be removed as soon as possible in order to provide relief or prevent

accidents or complications (e.g., agitation, combativeness, suicidal behavior); and

5. Understand the particular cognitive state of the delirious patient and factors that may influence it, in order to optimize nonspecific supportive measures in patient management (e.g., impaired capacity for information processing as influenced by an unfamiliar or ambiguous environment) (Balis, 1970; Sakles & Balis, 1978).

Etiologic Treatment

Every effort should be made to identify the underlying causative factor(s), with the aim of instituting specific treatment at the earliest possible time. A detailed history from relatives or friends is most helpful, especially in identifying drug ingestion, alcohol abuse, head trauma, chemical exposure, or already diagnosed disease (e.g., diabetes, epilepsy, drug idiosyncrasies, or heart disease). In hospitalized patients, the diagnostic process is aided by focusing on the setting in which the delirium occurred (I.C.U., recovery room, dialysis unit), the nature of preexisting disease (e.g., pulmonary insufficiency, cardiac failure, hepatic cirrhosis), or the nature of treatment of the primary disorder (e.g., digitalization, hypnotic–sedatives, continuous gastric suction, irradiation).

In view of the fact that the etiology of delirium is often multifactorial, especially in the hospitalized patient, the clinician should make an effort to search for several possible causative factors rather than a singular etiology. Although a single factor may cause delirium, several subthreshold factors acting concurrently may be sufficient to produce the critical physiological derangement that leads to the decompensated state. In this regard, every pathophysiological abnormality should be corrected and every possible etiologic factor eliminated, especially nonessential medications or those for which a less toxic drug can be substituted.

Once the causative factor is removed, the condition may be self-limited with rapid and complete recovery. In some instances, the primary cause may have already ceased to operate (e.g., head trauma, burns, seizures, bleeding, radiation) and only the pathogenic sequelae need to be treated (secondary causes). In others, the primary cause is unknown and only the disease processes are identifiable and amenable to treatment (e.g., effects of unknown drugs, fever of unknown origin). Sometimes all efforts fail to provide evidence of "organic" factors that might be related to a clinical delirium.

TABLE 2
Drugs Capable of Causing Delirium

Antidepressants (anticholinergic effect)

Neuroleptics (anticholinergic effect)

Antiparkinsonians (anticholinergic effect)

Anticholinergic/Antispasmodic
   atropine/homatropine
   belladonna alkaloids
   cyclopentolate (Cyclogyl)—eye drops
   scopolamine

Antihistamine (anticholinergic effect)
   brompheniramine (Dimetane)
   chlorpheniramine (Teldrin, Ornade)
   diphenhydramine (Benadryl)
   hydroxyzine (Vistaril, Atarax)
   promethazine (Phenergan)
   over-the-counter sleep and cold medicines

Anticonvulsant
   ethosuximide (Zarontin)
   phenytoin (Dilantin, others)
   primidone (Mysoline)
   sodium valprate (Depakene)

Sympathomimetic
   amphetamines
   ephedrine
   phenylephrine
   phenylpropanolamine
   phenetrazine
   diethylpropion
   methylphenidate (Ritalin)

Sedative–Hypnotic–Anxiolytic
   barbiturates
   glutethimide (Doriden)
   benzodiazepines
   meprobamate

Cardiovascular
   clonidine (Catapres)
   digitalis (Digoxin, Lanox)
   lidocaine (Xylocaine)
   methyldopa (Aldomet)
   propranolol (Inderal)
   procainamide (Pronestyl)
   quinidine (Quinidine, Duraquin)

(continued)

TABLE 2 *(continued)*

Miscellaneous
     amantadine (Symmetrel)
     aminocaproic acid (Amicar)
     aminophylline (Theo-Dur)
     amphotericin B (Fungizone)
     asparaginase (Wispar)
     baclofen (Lioresal)
     bromides
     carbidopa (Sinemet)
     chloroquine (Aralen)
     cimetidine (Tagamet)
     corticosteroids
     cortisones, prednisone, ACTH
     cycloserine (Seromycin)
     disulfiram (Antabuse)
     isoniazid
     ibuprofen (Motrin, Advil)
     indomethacin (Indocin)
     ketamine (Ketalar)
     levodopa (Dopar)
     lithium
     metrizamide (Amipaque)
     metronidazole (Flagyl)
     phenylbutazone (Butazolidin)
     naproxen (Naprosyn)
     quinacrine (Atabrine)
     theophylline
     5-fluorouracil

While searching for an etiologic diagnosis of the delirium, the clinician is called upon to recognize emergency situations presenting with delirium, either because they may be life-threatening or because of the possibility of irreversible brain damage (dementia) should the condition be prolonged. Early recognition and emergency treatment intervention reduce risk or degree of brain injury, general morbidity, and mortality. Common preventable etiologies associated with such risk include drug intoxication, hypoglycemia, diabetic acidosis, hypoxia or anoxia, thiamine deficiency, intracranial hemorrhage, subdural hematoma, subarachnoid or intracerebral hemorrhage due to ruptured aneurysm, withdrawal delirium, acute cerebral edema, and hyperthermia. Delirium as a complication of serious illness often portends life-threatening or ominous outcome.

Symptomatic Treatment

This is directed toward two areas: psychiatric symptoms of the delirium and the physical symptoms of the underlying disorder. Its purpose is to provide relief, improve morbidity, and prevent complications through an appropriately targeted approach to symptom control. Symptomatic treatment may be the only therapeutic approach available in those instances in which etiologic diagnosis is lacking.

The symptomatic treatment of the delirium is primarily medicinal. It should be emphasized, however, that the clinical picture of many delirious patients may not require any drug treatment other than general supportive management, and that appropriate management approaches may minimize or make unnecessary the use of drugs. For instance, when the clinical picture is characterized by a simple confusional state without symptoms of agitation, fear, or combativeness, medicinal treatment is unnecessary and may even be contraindicated since the psychotropic drugs that are commonly used for symptomatic relief may aggravate the delirium through their depressant, anticholinergic, or hypotensive effects (Heizer & Wilbert, 1974). Even in florid deliria in which the patient's emotional and behavioral reaction to the cognitive impairment dominates the clinical picture, pharmacologic control of symptoms should be judicious and tempered by the realization that appropriately supportive management measures may be of equal or even of greater importance.

Medicinal control of delirium generally involves the relief of distressing symptoms (fear, anxiety, panic, irritability, angry outbursts, illusory and hallucinatory symptoms, delusions) and disruptive behaviors (excitement, agitation, restlessness, combativeness, assaultiveness, hyperactivity, insomnia). Psychotropic drugs have no therapeutic effect on the cognitive deficit and, as mentioned earlier, may even worsen it. Physostigmine will restore cognitive functions in deliria induced by anticholinergic agents. Drugs recommended for the symptomatic control of delirious symptoms include antipsychotic (neuroleptic) and anxiolytic drugs (benzodiazepines). The choice of a particular psychotropic medication is based on several considerations including etiology of the delirium, biometabolism and side effects of the drug, and one's previous experience. Thorough familiarity with a drug's pharmacological actions, pharmacokinetics, biometabolism, and side effects enables the physician to tailor the treatment to the patient's particular needs.

High potency neuroleptics (haloperidol, perphenazine, thiothixene, fluphenazine, and trifluoperazine) show minimal sedative and autonomic (anticholinergic and alpha-blocking) effects, but a high incidence of extrapyramidal reactions (dystonia, akathesia, and parkinsonism). They are effective in the control of the delirious psychopathology including agitation, fear, and psychotic symptoms. The neuroleptic of choice in most cases is haloperidol (Ayd, 1978).

The anxiolytic benzodiazepines (chlordiazepoxide, diazepam, oxazepam, lorazepam, etc.) are safe and effective. They are less sedating than the hypnotics, require high doses to produce CNS depression, and have minimal autonomic action or effect on the cardiovascular and respiratory systems. They have a measurable anticonvulsant activity that may be useful in treating withdrawal deliria. They differ in pharmacokinetics and biometabolism, with oxazepam and lorazepam having a short plasma half-life, and chlordiazepoxide and diazepam lasting much longer. Oxazepam and lorazepam may therefore be the benzodiazepines of choice for treating patients expected to show cumulative effects (hepatic or renal insufficiency or prolonged use of the drug) (Lipowski, 1980a, b).

The prescription schedule of any of these drugs should also take into consideration the fluctuating course of delirium. If the timing of occurrence of the symptoms is characteristic (e.g., at night), it is advisable to prescribe the drug only prior to the onset of symptoms (Dubovsky & Weisberg, 1982).

The dosage and route of administration of these drugs depend on the severity of the symptoms, responsiveness to the drug, the patient's age (the elderly require much lower doses), and other factors. Small, preferably oral dosages are appropriate for moderate anxiety and restlessness. Higher doses, given parenterally, are required for the control of severe agitation, panic states, or assaultive behavior. The art of optimal titration of the drug, in order to be able to meet the changing needs of the delirious patient, requires close monitoring of therapeutic response and knowledge of all factors that may modify drug effects. Common problems associated with a failure to titrate the drug optimally include oversedation ("snowing" effect) resulting in stupor or even coma and respiratory depression, and undersedation with ineffective control of the symptoms.

When the choice of drug is haloperidol, the following approach is generally recommended. In mildly to moderately agitated patients, 2–10 mg given orally twice a day generally suffice. Parenteral administration might be necessary for the uncooperative patient, with the dosage adjusted to about three-fourths of the oral amount. In severely agitated, assaultive, or panicked patients, haloperidol should be given parenterally

(IM), with an initial dose of 2–10 mg, which can be repeated several times a day as needed, observing for adverse effects, until control of agitation is achieved (Lipowski, 1980a,b). The so-called "rapid neuroleptization method" has been suggested as a means of handling emergency situations and is described elsewhere. Doses should be lower than those for nonorganic disorders. The total daily dose required to produce a calming effect may range from 10–40 mg (or higher). Once this effect is achieved haloperidol should be given orally, in b.i.d. doses (Moore, 1977), and be gradually tapered and discontinued within days or weeks.

When benzodiazepines are used, the choice depends primarily on differences in their plasma half-lives and hepatic metabolism. In mildly to moderately agitated patients, 25–30 mg of chlordiazepoxide, 5–10 mg of diazepam, 15–30 mg of oxazepam, or 0.5–1.0 mg of lorazepam given orally every four to six hours as needed is generally sufficient. These doses may be doubled in more severely agitated patients. Parenteral (IM) administration of lorazepam may be required for patients showing severe agitation, panic, or combativeness, at dosage levels comparable to those for oral administration. In emergency situations, slow intravenous injection of chlordiazepoxide (25–50 mg) or diazepam (5–10 mg) may become necessary in order to bring the symptoms under immediate control.

Hydroxyzine, an antihistamine, and paraldehyde, a hypnotic, may also be used for control of anxiety and agitation, in a manner similar to that described for the benzodiazepines. Hydroxyzine may be given orally or parenterally, while paraldehyde is preferably administered rectally.

In addition to the symptomatic control of the psychiatric manifestations of delirium, close attention must be paid to correcting any concomitant pathophysiological derangement, even though not directly related to the primary etiology of the delirium. The symptomatic treatment may involve a broad range of disturbances including fever, insomnia, cardiac arrhythmias, seizures, dehydration, nutritional deficits, and urinary retention.

Patient Management
The management of the delirious patient in a hospital setting is the cornerstone of the total therapeutic approach. Its effectiveness is based on an understanding of the cognitive state of the patient and the factors that may influence it, as well as on an appreciation of the patient's psychological needs. Its goals are: (1) to optimize the patient's envi-

ronment and the staff's bedside approach as a means of providing support to the patient's cognitive deficit; (2) to provide protection from accidents; and (3) to improve and maintain the patient's physical and mental state through nonspecific supportive measures that provide control and comfort. The key for successful management is the quality of nursing care.

The primary physician must be thoroughly familiar with the management of the delirious patient in a hospital setting (Dubovsky & Weisberg, 1982). In managing a delirious patient, one should be guided by the awareness that the patient is confused and disoriented, has impaired memory and cannot retain new information, has difficulty processing information, tends to misinterpret events and distort their meaning, cannot tolerate either excessive or diminished sensory input, and may be experiencing perceptual distortions in the form of illusions or even hallucinations that are often frightening.

The patient with a mild delirium of known etiology and good prognosis (e.g., idiosyncratic reaction to a drug, febrile illness) is best cared for at home, within a stable and familiar environment, and under the continuous care and supervision of family members. Patients with more serious deliria, and especially those of unknown etiology, require immediate hospitalization. The choice of hospital type depends on several considerations, including etiology of the underlying illness, degree and sophistication of medical and diagnostic requirements, and severity of behavioral disturbances. For instance, patients with a delirium due to serious physical illness (e.g., heart failure) should be treated in a general hospital; in cases of alcohol withdrawal delirium, treatment may best be carried out in a detoxification unit; violent, suicidal, or acutely psychotic patients who show no evidence of serious physical illness require psychiatric hospitalization. Psychiatric consultation is required in most cases for assistance in diagnosis and management.

The physical environment should be stable and unambiguous, with elements that enhance familiarity and orientation, and maintain low sensory input, while at the same time preserving variability through stimulus change. The patient is best cared for in a quiet, simply furnished, and preferably single-bed room, softly lighted at all times, with mild stimulation provided by a radio or television set. A calendar, clock, and some personal articles (family pictures) should be at bedside for orientation and familiarity. Continuous supervision, preferably by a relative or friend who is thoroughly instructed about the requirements of this task, should be provided. Effort should be made to minimize the number of the nursing and house staff involved in the care of the patient, in order to increase the patient's familiarity with personnel. Special attention should be given to the overriding need for constant supervision and for instituting measures for protection from accidents, including suicidal and homicidal precautions when indicated. Physical restraints should be avoided whenever possible, and when applied they should be used for only brief periods. Control of agitation and combativeness is best managed by the personal contact of a supervising family member and by the appropriate use of tranquilizing drugs.

The interpersonal aspects of management are primarily determined by the patient's need to be oriented, to comprehend what is happening to him or her, and to be reassured. Accordingly, every interaction with the patient should adhere at all times to an approach that meets these needs. Professional staff should clearly identify themselves, state their role, remind the patient that he or she is in a hospital, and carefully explain what they intend to do. They should provide reassurance and explanation about everything that the patient experiences as alien, ambiguous, threatening, or frightening.

Upon recovery from the delirious state, the patient may have complete amnesia for the episode or may have spotty or incomplete recollection. If the patient is amnestic, he or she should be helped to understand the nature of the experiential gap and be reassured that his or her memory is now intact in spite of the amnesia. If the patient remembers the psychotic experiences (especially delusions and hallucinations), their nature and benign prognosis should be carefully explained.

SPECIFIC DELIRIA

The preceding section described the symptomatic treatment and management of delirium as an Organic Mental Syndrome (OMS), that is, without reference to etiology. *DSM–III–R* codes for deliria of unknown etiology include Axis I diagnoses when an unspecified psychoactive substance is suspected (292.81) and Axis III diagnoses for all other unknown etiologies (293.00).

The following section deals with specific treatments of deliria of known etiology. The previously described basic principles of symptomatic treatment and management of delirium are also applicable to these disorders. *DSM–III–R* classifies deliria of known etiology into three categories: (1) Psychoactive Substance-Induced Deliria; (2) Deliria Complicating Dementias Arising in the Senium and Presenium; and (3) Deliria Associated with Axis III Physical Disorders or Conditions.

1. Psychoactive Substance-Induced Deliria

These are most common and are generally associated with substance use disorders, suicidal or accidental drug overdose, and idiosyncratic reactions to prescribed or over-the-counter drugs. The pathogenic mechanism depends on the pharmacologic action(s) of the drug. Predisposing or facilitating factors include age (the elderly being most susceptible), biological substrate of the host (genetically determined enzyme systems), dosage, route of administration, hepatic function, and other (Balis, 1982). Clinically, these deliria can be classified into dose-related, idiosyncratic, and withdrawal types. This distinction allows definition of different approaches to treatment.

Dose-Related Deliria

These are deliria induced by relatively high blood concentrations of a potentially deliriogenic drug, such as certain psychoactive drugs (e.g., cocaine, amphetamines, phencyclidine) and anticholinergic agents. The major etiologic treatment approach is the elimination or inactivation by an antidote of the causative agent.

Idiosyncratic Deliria

These are not dose-related and can occur early in the course of treatment at therapeutic doses. Genetically controlled enzymatic processes in drug metabolism are thought to be responsible for the induction of the delirium (Balis, 1982). Many prescription drugs may cause idiosyncratic deliria in predisposed individuals (e.g., codeine, diazepam, glutethimide, chloroquine). They clear rapidly without any sequelae. Treatment is symptomatic.

Withdrawal Deliria

This is a special class of substance-induced deliria involving a different pathogenetic mechanism, as well as different *DSM-III-R* coding. These deliria occur in individuals who have developed physiological dependence on alcohol (291.00) or sedative–hypnotic–anxiolytic drugs (292.00), usually following prolonged use, during withdrawal from the agent. Their treatment is discussed in the section on Withdrawal and Withdrawal Deliria in Chapter 12.

The *DSM-III-R* lists on Axis I the following specific psychoactive substance-induced deliria, under the code 292.81.

292.81 Cocaine Delirium

Cocaine-induced delirium may develop in both the naive and the chronic cocaine user. The syndrome occurs almost immediately following intravenous injection or smoking ("free-basing"), usually within one hour (but not more than 24 hours) of intake of cocaine. In uncomplicated cases, the delirium clears within six hours. Its treatment is similar to that of intoxication with psychostimulant drugs (see Intoxications in Chapter 12). The patient requires placement in a quiet room where safety measures (e.g., physical restraints) may be applied for the protection of the combative individual. Agitation can be controlled by the use of benzodiazepines (e.g., lorazepam 1 mg IM q 2–4 hours prn) or neuroleptics (e.g., haloperidol 5 mg IM or 5–15 mg po q 2–4 hours prn). It should be noted, however, that cocaine abusers may be sensitive to the extrapyramidal side effects of the neuroleptics because of dopamine depletion (Perry, 1987). The patient's vital signs should be monitored very closely for rising temperature, pulse, and blood pressure. Hyperthermia (above 29°C) requires vigorous treatment with both hypothermic blankets and ice packs to prevent grand mal seizures. If convulsions do occur, the patient should be treated with slowly administered intravenous diazepam 5–15 mg q 15 to 45 minutes to prevent progression to status epilepticus. Uncontrollable severe hypertension (systolic blood pressure remaining above 200 mg Hg for an hour or more) should be controlled promptly with propranolol (Perry, 1987).

292.81 Amphetamine or Similarly Acting Sympathomimetic Delirium

Sympathomimetic drugs with a CNS stimulant action include, besides amphetamine, cocaine, methylphenidate (Ritalin) and diethylpropion (Tenuate). All these psychostimulant drugs may induce delirium within 24 hours of intake, and almost immediately following intravenous administration. In addition to confusional symptoms, associated features include tactile and olfactory hallucinations, labile affect, and violent behavior. The patient needs to be closely monitored for rising blood pressure and temperature and occurrence of convulsions. Treatment of psychostimulant delirium is similar to that of Cocaine Delirium and psychostimulant intoxication.

292.81 Phencyclidine (PCP) or Similarly Acting Arylcyclohexylamine Delirium

The delirium may develop within 24 hours after intake or it may emerge days later after recovery from an overdose. It may last for a week with a waxing and waning course. Associated features are those of phencyclidine intoxication including both physiological changes (e.g., ataxia, dysarthria, muscular rigidity, nystagmus, seizures, elevated blood pressure) and behavioral disturbances (e.g., fluctuations in mood, impulsivity, agitation, assaultiveness).

Treatment is similar to that described in the section of Phencyclidine Intoxication. It includes the provision of a calm environment and adequate restraints for combative behavior, and the use of diazepam or haloperidol for controlling agitation. If seizures develop, diazepam should be given intravenously to prevent status epilepticus. If serious hypertension develops, diazoxide and hydrazine have been reported to be effective in lowering blood pressure (Lewis & Senay, 1981).

292.81   Deliria Associated with Other Psychoactive Substance

Numerous drugs with psychoactive action (CNS effects) may induce delirium as a result of drug idiosyncrasy in predisposed individuals (genetically determined) or altered drug metabolism (e.g., elderly, impaired hepatic function, drug interaction), or because of toxic blood concentrations of the drug (e.g., overdose, cumulative effects, impaired renal excretion). Table 2 (pp. 61–62) lists drugs that are known to cause delirium. Many of these drugs possess an anticholinergic action. An anticholinergic mechanism is implicated in the majority of drug-induced deliria.

Anticholinergic Substance Delirium

Drugs with anticholinergic activity include many antispasmodics (atropine, homatropine, belladonna alkaloids, scopolamine, etc.), antiparkinsonians (benztropine, trihexyphenidyl, biperiden, etc.) analgesics (meperidine), tricyclic antidepressants (especially amitriptyline), neuroleptics (low potency, and especially thioridazine), antihistamines (diphenhydramine, promethazine, etc.), hydroxyzine, cimetidine, and others.

Tricyclic drug overdose is a common cause of anticholinergic delirium. According to Preskorn and Simpson (1982), tricyclic plasma levels exceeding 450 ng/ml produced delirium in six of seven patients. Delirium may also occur as an idiosyncratic phenomenon with blood concentrations within the therapeutic range (Godwin, 1983). The elderly are particularly vulnerable to anticholinergic delirium.

Treatment of anticholinergic delirium is similar to that described in the section on Anticholinergic Drug Intoxication. Physostigmine salicylate 1–2 mg IV or IM will clear the delirium within less than 30 minutes. A second dose of 1–2 mg physostigmine may be given 15 minutes later, and may be repeated every two to three hours if needed (Blitt & Petty, 1975; Eisendrath et al., 1987; Godwin, 1983; Heizer &

Wilbert, 1974; Lewis & Senay, 1981; Mogelnicki, Waller, & Finlayson, 1979; Perry, 1987).

In the case of anticholinergic delirium induced by tri- and tetracyclic antidepressants, one needs to monitor the EKG closely and treat, if necessary, the cardiotoxic effects of these drugs.

2. Deliria Complicating Dementias of the Senium and Presenium
The *DSM–III–R* Axis I provides the following codes for delirium complicating dementias:

> 290.30 Primary Degenerative Dementia of the Alzheimer Type, Senile Onset, with Delirium
> 290.11 Primary Degenerative Dementia of the Alzheimer Type, Presenile Onset with Delirium
> 290.41 Multi-infarct Dementia with Delirium

Delirium is one of the complicating syndromes often superimposed upon a dementia. This syndrome is also known as "acute confusional state." The etiology of these deliria is not uniform, and is generally not related directly to the pathogenic mechanism of the dementia itself. Most of them are drug-induced, often having an anticholinergic mechanism (see Table 2). Other etiologies include metabolic disorders (diabetic acidosis, or hypoglycemia, hepatic and renal insufficiency), hypoxia–anoxia resulting from cardiac or pulmonary disease, and other conditions listed in Table 1. One of the etiologies of delirium complicating Multi-infarct Dementia is the disease process itself, which may result in delirium during transient ischemic attacks (TIAs) and during the acute phase of an occlusive episode secondary to thrombosis or cerebral emboli (small stroke). Acute confusional episodes in the demented elderly that are characterized by transient, delirium-like cognitive disturbances judged to be functional and referred to as "pseudodelirium" by analogy with "pseudodementia" are particularly interesting (Lipowski, 1983). They generally occur in the evening or at night in the form of "sundowner" syndrome, as a result of diminished sensory input and social isolation and/or exposure to an unfamiliar environment (e.g., the hospital). The treatment of the "sundowner" syndrome consists of better orientation, room lights, and of small doses of a high potency neuroleptic (e.g., haloperidol 0.5 to 1 mg) given one or two hours before sundown. The dosage may be gradually increased as needed (DuBovsky & Weisberg, 1982).

290.30   Primary Degenerative Dementia of the Alzheimer Type, Senile Onset with Delirium

290.11   Primary Degenerative Dementia of the Alzheimer Type, Presenile Onset with Delirium

As with other deliria, therapy of delirium in the demented patient suffering from Alzheimer's disorder is both etiologic and symptomatic/ supportive. It consists of treatment or removal of the putative deliriogenic condition, while providing symptomatic therapy for agitation, psychotic symptoms, or insomnia, as well as supportive management through good nursing (Bayne, 1978; Lipowski, 1980a, 1983; Liston, 1982; Seymour et al., 1980; Wolanin & Phillips, 1981).

For control of agitation, high potency neuroleptics are recommended, and especially haloperidol in doses 0.5–5 mg po or IM twice daily (Lipowski, 1980b, 1983). If the patient develops intolerable extrapyramidal symptoms, agitation may be alternatively controlled with small doses of a short-half-life benzodiazepine, such as lorazepam (Ativan), which can be given in doses 0.5–1 mg po or IM q 4 to 6 hours prn. If insomnia is present, it may be treated with a short-half-life benzodiazepine hypnotic, such as temazepam (Restoril) 15–30 mg hs prn, or triazolam (Halcion). The clinician should keep in mind that the use of sedative/hypnotics and benzodiazepines, especially those with longer half-life (e.g., flurazepam, diazepam) may worsen the confusion in delirium, especially in the elderly, as a result of drug accumulation. For more information, see section on Dementia (p. 76).

290.41   Multi-infarct Dementia with Delirium

The development of delirium in a patient with multiple infarct dementia is a serious complication because of the patient's poor general health (hypertension, arteriosclerotic heart disease) and because of the possibility that the disease process itself may be causing the delirium as a result of transient ischemic attacks (TIAs) or thrombotic episodes in evolution. The latter etiology requires careful diagnostic evaluation before etiological treatment is instituted, in an effort to abort an irreversible cerebrovascular accident.

TIAs referable to the carotid or vertebrobasilar arterial territories may present with acute confusional symptoms constituting a delirium. TIAs last from a few seconds up to 12 hours and may occur repeatedly, leaving no sequelae or progressing to a thrombotic episode in the form of a small or catastrophic stroke. The treatment of TIAs consists of anticoagulants, aspirin, and vasodilators. Anticoagulant therapy (heparin, warfarin) may prevent TIAs and postpone an impending stroke. Anticoagulants may also arrest the advance of a thrombotic stroke-in-evolution. The use of anticoagulant drugs makes an accurate diagnosis imperative, especially in ruling out intracranial hemorrhage. Other measures that have been used in the treatment of TIAs include aspirin, cerebral vasodilators such as papaverine, nicotinic acid, inhalation of 5% carbon dioxide, aminophylline, and acetazolamide. The use of vasodilators is controversial and of questionable value. On the other hand, the prophylactic use of aspirin is generally recommended.

In the case of a thrombotic episode in evolution, anticoagulation with heparin IV or continuous drip therapy is instituted for several days, followed by oral warfarin at doses sufficient to maintain prothrombin time at twice the control value (Hass, 1979; Mohr et al., 1977). Currently used thrombolytic agents (e.g., fibrinolysin and pro-fibrinolysin activator) have not proved helpful in treating thrombosis-in-evolution (Mohr et al., 1977).

The treatment of deliria of other etiologies that occur in patients with multi-infarct dementia is similar to that described in the general section on Delirium.

3. Deliria Associated With Axis III Physical Disorders or Conditions

Most of the disorders listed in Table 1 may cause delirium, coded as 293.00. Metabolic disorders, systemic and CNS infections, head trauma, and postictal states are common etiologies and are listed in Axis III. Deliria of particular interest include Wernicke's encephalopathy and Neuroleptic Malignant Syndrome (NMS).

Wernicke's Syndrome

This acute encephalopathy is produced by nutritional deficiency involving thiamine, usually secondary to chronic alcoholism. Other conditions leading to Wernicke's syndrome include chronic hemodialysis, thyrotoxicosis, pernicious vomiting of pregnancy, and gastric carcinoma. It usually begins abruptly as a "quiet delirium" and is accompanied by characteristic neurologic signs that include external ophthalmoplegia, nystagmus, and cerebellar ataxia, as well as polyneuropathy. The patient most often appears apathetic, listless, confused, and disoriented.

Treatment of the syndrome consists of parenteral thiamine (50 mg IM) followed by oral doses of thiamine and good nutrition with multivitamin supplement. The ophthalmoplegia and signs of delirium show dramatic improvement within hours and clear completely within a few days after administration of thiamine. Nystagmus and ataxia improve more slowly. The patient emerges from the delirium several days later with an organic amnestic syndrome (Korsakoff's) (Victor, Adams, & Collins, 1971).

Neuroleptic Malignant Syndrome (NMS)

This syndrome presents unpredictably among psychiatric patients as an idiosyncratic response to therapeutic doses of neuroleptics. It is more likely to occur with high potency neuroleptics, especially when given parenterally, and in conjunction with lithium and other drugs. Dehydration and exhaustion are thought to be predisposing factors. In the author's opinion NMS appears to be a state-dependent response to neuroleptics often associated with excitement and agitation. It is thought to be the result of a neuroleptic-induced massive blockade of dopamine (DA) receptors, especially in the striatal, mesofrontal, and hypothalamic DA systems.

Clinically, the patient presents with catatonic-like symptoms of mutism, bradykinesia, and plastic (lead-type) rigidity with counterpull resistance (described by Kleist, 1936, as *Gegenhalten*), suggestive of frontal lobe involvement (mesofrontal DA blockade); often with cogwheel rigidity (basal ganglia DA blockade); autonomic dysregulation manifested by marked diaphoresis, tachycardia, fluctuating blood pressure (hypothalamic DA blockade); hypermetabolic state manifested by pyrexia, elevated serum CPK, leukocytosis, elevated liver enzymes, and cardiac arrhythmias (hypothalamic DA blockade); and confusional symptoms of a waxing and waning course, characteristic of delirium.

Symptoms typically resolve within five to 10 days or longer if depot neuroleptics were used (e.g., fluphenazine decanoate). Complications include rhabdomyolysis with myoglobulinemia resulting in acute renal failure, aspiration pneumonia, and cardiovascular collapse. Mortality has been estimated at 20% (Karoff, 1980; Levenson, 1985; Smego & Durack, 1982).

There are notable similarities between NMS and *postanesthetic malignant hyperthermia* (MH). The latter is due to a peripheral mechanism related to an idiopathic dysfunction in sarcoplasmic calcium-ion metabolism resulting in a hypermetabolic state of skeletal muscles (Nelson & Flewellen, 1983). *Lethal catatonia* may also mimic NMS.

The patient is best managed in a general hospital. Placement in I.C.U. may often become necessary during the course of the syndrome.

Treatment of NMS is essentially supportive, consisting of early recognition, immediate discontinuation of neuroleptic medications, and careful attention to the detection and aggressive management of complications: for example, control of hyperthermia with antipyretics and cooling blankets, correction of dehydration and electrolyte imbalance, treatment of intercurrent infection such as pneumonia; dialysis for acute renal failure following rhabdomyolysis; ventilator support in case of acute respiratory failure due to aspiration, infection, or pulmonary emboli; treatment of cardiac arrhythmias; and management of other secondary complications. Since the patient is usually immobile, prophylactic low-dose heparin has been suggested to prevent venous thrombosis and embolic episodes.

Various specific treatments have been advocated in case reports but their efficacy remains unclear. These include anticholinergics, dopamine agonists (e.g., bromocriptine and amantadine), dantrolene, lorazepam, and ECT. The data so far seem to support most strongly the use of bromocriptine and dantrolene. Bromocriptine, a dopamine agonist, has been used in dosages ranging from 7.5–60 mg/day, in divided doses every eight hours, intravenously at the beginning (Dhib-Jalbut et al., 1983; Granato et al., 1983; Mueller, Vester, & Fermaglich, 1983; Zubenko & Pope, 1983). Amantadine, another dopamine agonist, has been used in doses of 100 mg b.i.d. with some anecdotal success (Amdurski et al., 1983; McCarron, Boettger, & Peck, 1982).

Dantrolene has been the most frequently tried; it is a direct-acting muscle relaxant affecting calcium release from the sarcoplasmic reticulum, and used successfully in treating malignant hyperthermia. It has been used in NMS in a dose range of 0.8–2.5 mg/kg every six hours (oral regimens ranged from 100–300 mg/daily in divided doses for two to three days) (Coons, Hillman, & Marshall, 1982; Goekoop & Carbaat, 1982; Kahn et al., 1985; May et al., 1983; Zubenko & Pope, 1983). Anticholinergic agents have not been found to be useful (Karoff, 1980; Levenson, 1985). ECT has been reported to be useful but may result in lethal cardiac arrhythmias (Jessee & Anderson, 1983). Lorazepam may be a safe and useful drug (Fricchione et al., 1983). Further experience is necessary before routinely recommending these agents. Reintroduction of neuroleptics in post-NMS cases must be done very cautiously, preferably with a low potency neuroleptic to avoid possible recurrence of the syndrome (Mueller, Vester, & Fermaglich, 1983; Scarlett, Zimmerman, & Berkovic, 1983). Although NMS cases have been reported to resolve without residual symptoms, the writer has noted two cases followed by permanent brain damage manifested as severe frontal lobe syndrome with catatonic-like symptoms, severe perseveration, gait disturbance, and dementia.

10B: DEMENTIA

The term *dementia,* as currently used, does not carry the prognostic connotation of a progressive or irreversible course implied in the past. Depending on the underlying organic etiology, dementia may be reversible or irreversible. Its clinical course may be progressive, static, or remitting. Most of the causes of Organic Mental Disorders listed in Table 1 may produce dementia, either as a primary disorder (e.g., Primary Degenerative [Alzheimer's type] Dementia) or as a secondary disorder, often progressing from an initial phase of delirium (e.g., protracted cerebral hypoxia, hypoglycemia).

The differential diagnosis of reversible dementias is of great prognostic significance. Early diagnosis of these disorders is of utmost importance. Dementia must be differentiated from delirium (no clouding of consciousness in dementia), Amnestic Syndrome (deficit involves only memory), and from the so-called "pseudodementia," a form of depression masquerading as dementia, which must always be ruled out before the diagnosis is made (Caine, 1981).

General Therapeutic Principles

The following general guidelines apply to the treatment and management of all dementias, with special emphasis on those arising in the senium. Treatment may be etiologic (when the cause is known and treatable) and/or symptomatic.

Etiologic Treatment

In searching for a treatable cause, first consideration should be given to ruling out depressive pseudodementia. A trial treatment with antidepressants may be justified in the absence of demonstrable etiology. The next step is to search for possible treatable organic causes (Cummings, Benson, & LoVerme, 1980), especially when an etiologic diagnosis remains uncertain. This is particularly important in older patients, who are more likely to be diagnosed as suffering from Alzheimer's disease or Multi-infarct Dementia, often in the absence of any objective evidence. A diagnostic battery for screening etiologically treatable dementias often includes the following tests (McAllister & Price, 1982; Wells, 1979):

- Serology test for syphilis
- Complete blood count
- Serum B12, folate, T3 or T4
- Urinalysis
- Metabolic screen
- Drug screen
- Computerized axial tomography (CT-scan)

Additional examination and laboratory procedures may be needed (e.g., magnetic resonance imaging [MRI], serum electrolytes, HIV screening [for high-risk persons]).

Symptomatic Treatment

This is the only therapeutic approach available for those patients suffering from irreversible forms of dementia. Since the cognitive deficit of irreversible dementia is not amenable to any treatment, all therapeutic efforts are directed toward improving impaired functions, promoting general health, and treating psychiatric complications when they develop.

Demented patients, especially the elderly, must maintain the best possible physical health in order to prevent the consequences of physiological derangement of their already compromised cerebral functions. Every effort should be made to restore or improve impaired physical functions (e.g., renal, cardiovascular, respiratory, or endocrine), combat symptoms (pain, insomnia, constipation, impaired mobility), improve impaired hearing and vision, and maintain an optimal nutritional state.

The prevention of toxic effects of medication, prescribed or over-the-counter, is of particular importance, especially those resulting from drug interactions. Elderly patients are particularly susceptible to side effects because of decreased physiologic reserves and slower rates of absorption, metabolism, and elimination of many drugs (Salzman, Shader, & Pearlman, 1970). Demented patients are highly vulnerable to the development of secondary psychiatric disorders, including delirium, depression, and psychosis. The following is a brief review of the treatment of some common psychiatric problems in dementia.

Insomnia. This is a ubiquitous complaint of the elderly. Demented patients often cannot fall asleep as a result of becoming disoriented and frightened when the lights are turned out. The first measure to recommend is leaving a light on all night. Patients with sleep-onset insomnia may benefit from L-tryptophan, which can be prescribed as a pill or provided through high tryptophan foods such as milk or tuna fish.

When drug treatment becomes necessary, antihistamines in low doses are well tolerated (e.g., promethazine hydrochloride 25–50 mg or diphenhydramine 25–50 mg at bedtime) (Salzman, 1982). Antihistamines at higher doses may induce anticholinergic delirium. Thioridazine 25 mg is also effective and well tolerated. Chloral hydrate in doses 250–500 mg is recommended as the next least toxic drug. The hypnotic benzodiazepines (e.g., flurazepam, triazolam, temazepam), although the most widely prescribed hypnotics, work only for a few weeks, and the longer half-life ones (e.g., flurazepam) tend to produce unwanted daytime drowsiness, ataxia, and confusion. Insomnia secondary to another disorder (e.g., depression) should be treated etiologically.

Anxiety. Benzodiazepines are the drugs of choice for treating nonpsychotic anxiety states when psychological approaches fail to control the symptoms. In choosing a suitable benzodiazepine for the elderly demented patient, the clinician must take into consideration the kinetics and biotransformation of the various representatives of this class of anxiolytics (see Symptomatic Treatment section on Delirium). The long-acting chlordiazepoxide and diazepam are undesirable because of cumulative effects. The short-acting oxazepam and lorazepam are preferred, prescribed in approximately one-third to one-half of the younger adult dose. Excessive sedation, apathy, ataxia, incoordination, disorientation, confusion, and dysarthria are common toxic effects (Salzman, 1982).

Agitation. Restlessness, wandering around, and agitation are commonly seen in elderly demented patients. These symptoms tend to be more severe in the evening and at night ("sundowner syndrome") and are often part of a psychosis. Neuroleptics have been shown to be effective. In a recent review by Salzman (1987), neuroleptics show a therapeutic response of "good to excellent" in 60%–70% of elderly agitated patients with a wide variety of organic and emotional disorders. No therapeutic differences among neuroleptics can be inferred.

Delirium. This is the most common psychiatric complication, especially in patients with Multi-infarct Dementia. Various drugs, especially anticholinergic, are very common causes of delirium in the elderly. For treatment, see section on Delirium.

Depression. Treatment of depression includes various psychotherapeutic approaches, antidepressant medication, and ECT (Ban, 1987b; Butler, 1975). In milder forms of dementia, supportive psychotherapy is useful in assisting the patient to grieve and accept cognitive losses and their consequences, and to maintain self-esteem. Psychotherapeutic management approaches are directed toward enhancing environmental–social support throughout the course of dementia.

In the presence of severe depression, tri- or tetracyclic antidepressants have been the preferred drugs. The choice of a specific tricyclic depends on clinical considerations as modified by the altered metabolism of the elderly (Hrdina et al., 1980; Robinson, 1979). Several side effects of the tricyclics are especially hazardous for the elderly, because aging increases plasma half-life and steady-state plasma levels, especially with imipramine and amitriptyline. Side effects include sedation, orthostatic hypotension, anticholinergic effects, and cardiotoxicity.

The higher sedating effects of certain tricyclics (amitriptyline, doxepin) may be desirable in some patients for controlling insomnia, with two-thirds or more of the daily dose given before bedtime. The hypotensive effect of tricyclics does not seem to increase with advancing age (Glassman et al., 1979; Roose et al., 1981); nevertheless, orthostatic hypotension is a very common side effect and may precipitate falls, strokes, or heart attacks. Nortriptyline, compared with imipramine, produces less hypotension (Roose et al., 1981).

Anticholinergic activity is especially prominent with amitriptyline, while desipramine, and to a lesser extent nortriptyline, have the least anticholinergic action. Trazodone has little or none. Elderly demented patients are particularly vulnerable to CNS anticholinergic toxicity, with one-third of patients on tricyclics being reported to develop confusion or delirium (Davies et al., 1971). Cardiotoxicity is of particular concern; tricyclics may produce sinus tachycardia, prolonged intraventricular conduction, and probably decreased myocardial contractility, as well as arrhythmias (Bigger et al., 1978). Imipramine appears to have antiarrhythmic properties.

In view of the above, the tricyclics of choice are desipramine, nortriptyline, and doxepin. Of the three, desipramine is the least anticholinergic, and doxepin the least cardiotoxic (Salzman, 1982; Salzman et al., 1970). The so-called second generation antidepressants (e.g., maprotiline, amoxapine, trazodone) are reported to have fewer anticholinergic and cardiovascular side effects and therefore may present some advantage over the older tricyclics in the treatment of the elderly patient, a claim which has not been well documented (Gerner et al.,

1980). The recently introduced fluoxetine Hcl (Prozac) may prove to be a better tolerated alternative.

The following general guidelines apply in prescribing tricyclic drugs for the elderly demented patient:

1. Obtain a pretreatment electrocardiogram and repeat ECG periodically during course of treatment.
2. Measure seated and standing blood pressure before treatment is started and before each increase in dose.
3. Start with very low doses (e.g., 20–40 mg, imipramine equivalent, daily in divided doses) and raise dose gradually, monitoring both therapeutic response and side effects (50–150 mg, imipramine equivalent, per day is the usual therapeutic range).
4. Give two-thirds of the dose before bedtime to promote sleep.
5. The concurrent administration of volume-depleting diuretics increases risk of orthostatic hypotension.
6. Exercise extreme caution in patients with preexisting cardiovascular disease and patients receiving quinidine or procainamide, and be fully familiar with contraindicated drug combinations (clonidine, guanethidine, or bethanidine).
7. Monitor tricyclic plasma levels regularly, in order to prevent cumulative toxic levels (Salzman, 1982).

Monoamine oxidase inhibitors (MAOIs), such as phenelzine (Nardil) and tranylcypromine (Parnate), have been shown to be effective antidepressants, which are safe and well tolerated by the elderly (Jenike, 1985). Their major advantage over the tricyclics is that they lack anticholinergic and cardiotoxic effects.

Electroconvulsive therapy (ECT) may be indicated in depressed demented patients without posterior fossa space-occupying lesions who fail to respond to an adequate course of antidepressants and patients who cannot tolerate the side effects or adverse effects of tricyclics or MAOIs (Salzman, 1975).

Psychosis. Psychotic symptoms are amenable to treatment with neuroleptic drugs, which, although equally effective in controlling psychotic thinking and behavior, differ in side effects and toxicity (Hamilton, 1966). As with the tricyclics, the choice of a specific antipsychotic agent should be based on considerations regarding toxicity and altered metabolism in the elderly (Salzman, 1982, 1987). Common side effects of neuroleptic drugs which may have serious consequences include sedation, orthostatic hypotension, anticholinergic effects, and extrapyramidal symptoms. Impaired thermoregulation and idiosyncratic reactions should also be noted.

Although the sedative effects of neuroleptics may be used therapeutically to induce sleep at night or tranquilize the agitated patient during daytime, they often produce confusion and disorientation in the elderly. Low potency neuroleptics (chlorpromazine, thioridazine, mesoridazine, chlorprothixene) have the strongest sedative effects, while the high potency neuroleptics (haloperidol, fluphenazine, perphenazine, trifluoperazine, thiothixene) are least sedative. Low potency neuroleptics also have the strongest autonomic effects (hypotensive and anticholinergic) but show fewer extrapyramidal side effects. Conversely, high potency neuroleptics have minimal autonomic effects but very frequent extrapyramidal side effects.

Although high potency neuroleptics are generally safer and the drugs of choice for patients in whom autonomic and sedative effects are most hazardous, low potency neuroleptics (e.g., thioridazine) in small doses may be more appropriate for restless and agitated psychotic patients and those who are sensitive to extrapyramidal reactions (Steele, Lucas, & Tune, 1986). Elderly demented patients are particularly susceptible to orthostatic hypotension (Blumenthal & Davie, 1980), as well as to central anticholinergic toxicity (confusion, delirium) and extrapyramidal effects (Raskind & Risse, 1986; Salzman, 1982; Salzman et al., 1970). Neuroleptic treatment should begin with small amounts of the medication, given in divided doses (e.g., haloperidol 0.5–2 mg daily, or thioridazine 25–75 mg daily).

Patient Management

Effective management of the demented patient demands commitment on the part of the physician to accepting the responsibility for continuing care to a chronically ill and, in most instances, progressively deteriorating patient (Plutzky, 1974). The traditional medical model is expanded to include additional roles required for dealing with social and family problems confronting the patient and his or her caretakers.

The physician is often called upon to coordinate the activities of several caregivers including family members, social workers, visiting nurses, in-house aides, and other social service personnel. Knowledge of available community resources and how they can be utilized in the total care of the demented patient is a prerequisite. Knowledge of the patient's medical and psychological needs, family resources and interpersonal dynamics, assets and liabilities, prognosis, and anticipated problems are all crucial for treatment planning.

The physician should maintain continuing interaction with family members, inform them about the patient's condition, advise them about property management, and involve them in the patient's treatment. He or she should also provide emotional support and assist with their feelings of shame, guilt, or anger, especially when they must make decisions about institutional placement of the patient. Relatives often become highly critical of the physician or nursing home staff as a means of coping with feelings of guilt or helplessness. These reactions can be prevented or resolved through ventilation and moral support.

The doctor–patient relationship should remain a significant focus through the course of the illness. This is most important earlier in progressive dementias and in those patients with nonprogressive dementias, such as those which follow an acute brain insult (e.g., head trauma, encephalitis, anoxia, and hypoglycemic syndromes). The physician should structure each visit with the patient to provide psychological support by allaying fears, counteracting the sense of helplessness, allowing ventilation of feelings, enhancing self-esteem, encouraging independence, strengthening healthier coping mechanisms, and correcting distortions of reality when present.

Rehabilitation through retraining is needed for those patients with milder residual deficit and nonprogressive dementias. Every effort should be made to maintain ambulation and prevent regression to wheelchair or bed. Other guidelines in the management of the demented patient include encouragement of efforts toward maximum feasible independence and self-care; engagement in pleasurable, useful, or productive activities that enhance self-esteem; maintenance of preserved skills and abilities, as well as physical fitness; and appropriate supervision to prevent consequences of poor memory (e.g., fire hazards, getting lost, poor nutrition, deterioration of personal hygiene) or impaired social judgment (e.g., poor management of financial matters and personal affairs).

Appropriate manipulation of the patient's physical environment, whether in an institution or at home, is an important means of supporting impaired cognitive function, such as memory and orientation, and impaired sensory perception. Environmental modulation to establish a "prosthetic environment" for the demented patient includes good room lighting; simple, stable, and familiar furnishings; clocks that sound the time and large calendars on the wall; note pads as memory aids; pill boxes; hearing aids; eyeglasses; dentures; handrails; a walker, and so forth.

SPECIFIC DEMENTIAS

The preceding section dealt with the nonspecific, symptomatic treatment of Dementia without reference to etiology. *DSM–III–R* codes for dementia of unknown etiology include Axis I diagnoses when an unspecified psychoactive substance is suspected (292.82) and Axis III diagnoses for all other unknown etiologies (294.10). The following section discusses specific treatments of dementia of known etiology. The previously described basic principles of symptomatic treatment and supportive management of dementia are also applicable to these disorders.

From a clinical standpoint (prognostic and therapeutic) it is useful to classify dementias into these which are irreversible and reversible.

Irreversible dementias are associated with permanent neuronal damage and may be (a) progressive or (b) residual (nonprogressive). *Progressive dementias* have a relentless course toward a vegetative state and death. They include Primary Degenerative Dementia of the Alzheimer type (Senile and Presenile Onset), Multi-infarct Dementia, and other less common disorders such as Huntington's chorea, progressive supranuclear palsy, and Parkinson's disease. *Residual (nonprogressive) dementias* include those secondary dementias resulting from cerebral trauma, protracted cerebral hypoxia or hypoglycemia, and other permanent but nonprogressive injuries to the brain. The latter are of great clinical significance because the underlying cerebral disorder can be prevented, arrested, or fully reversed or eliminated if appropriate etiologic treatment is applied early (Cummings, Benson, & LoVerme, 1980).

Reversible dementias are syndromes with a treatable underlying organic disorder. They are of great significance prognostically and therapeutically. The substance-induced dementias (e.g., bromides, barbiturates, steroids), for example, are eminently treatable. The *DSM–III–R* classifies dementias of known etiology into the following categories: (1) Dementias Arising in the Senium and Presenium (290.XX); (2) Psychoactive Substance-Induced Dementias (291.20, 292.82); and (3) Dementias Associated with Axis III Physical Disorders or Conditions (294.10).

1. Dementias Arising in the Senium and Presenium
290.xx   Primary Degenerative Dementia of the Alzheimer Type, Senile Onset
290.1x   Primary Degenerative Dementia of the Alzheimer Type, Presenile Onset

These are the most common dementias in the elderly, affecting 7% of the population over 65 years of age and accounting for 25%–30% of all cases of dementia (Cummings, 1987; Cummings & Benson, 1983). The dementia begins insidiously and progresses slowly, first with symptoms of memory loss followed by progressive intellectual impairment and personality changes, and later with symptoms of aphasia and apraxia, finally reaching a vegetative state after 8–10 years or longer (Reisberg et al., 1987). Compared to patients with Multi-infarct Dementia, patients with Alzheimer's dementia seem to enjoy relatively good physical health.

The etiology of this neurodegenerative disorder remains unknown. Some cases appear to have a familial occurrence (Heston et al., 1981). Recent advances in the neurochemistry of Alzheimer's disease have revealed striking neurotransmitter changes and characteristic cellular proteins (Davies & Wolozin, 1987). Acetylcholine deficit is of particular research and clinical interest, as shown by loss of cortical markers of the cholinergic system: for example, decreased choline acetyltransferase (Davies & Maloney, 1976; Perry et al., 1977), loss of the cholinergic neurons in the nucleus basalis of Meynert (Whitehouse et al., 1982), and decrease of M2 muscarinic receptors (Mash, Flynn, & Potter, 1985).

Apparently, the ventral forebrain cholinergic neurons projecting to the cerebral cortex and hippocampus are the most consistently and severely damaged. Using monoclonal antibodies to ventral forebrain tissue from patients who died with Alzheimer's disease, Wolozin et al. (1986) identified a protein, Az-50, which is an interesting marker of Alzheimer's disease.

On the evidence of a cholinergic deficit associated with Alzheimer's dementia, a number of studies have tested the therapeutic efficacy of the available cholinomimetic drugs. So far, efforts to reverse or arrest cognitive deficit with the use of acetylcholine agonists or precursors have failed to provide significant results. Choline and phosphatidyl choline (PhosChol), dietary precursors of acetylcholine, have been found to be ineffective in improving the cognitive deficit (Thal et al., 1981), probably because these substances do not substantially affect cholinergic activity.

Clinical trials with I.V. physostigmine indicate transient enhancement of memory performance of patients with Alzheimer's disease (Christie et al., 1981; Davis et al., 1982). One major disadvantage of this drug, besides its side effects, is its plasma half-life of only about 30 minutes. Oral physostigmine in doses of 2 mg every two hours for several days was found to be beneficial (Mohs et al., 1985).

Available long-acting cholinesterase inhibitors and cholinergic agonists such as isoflurophate and oxotremorine, respectively, have potentially serious toxicity. Oral tetrahydroaminoacridine (THA), a centrally active anticholinesterase, was recently found by Summers et al. (1986)

in preliminary long-term trials to produce significant cognitive improvement. Several controlled studies using THA are currently under way. There is some interest in studying the efficacy of the so-called nootropic drugs, such as piracetam, and ACTH-4-10 (Cole & Braconnier, 1980; Reisberg, Ferris, & Gershon, 1981; Salzman, 1979), as well as intravenous naloxone (Reisberg et al., 1982).

Numerous other drugs have been used in the treatment of Alzheimer's dementia with questionable results, including central nervous system stimulants (e.g., pentylenetetrazol, amphetamines, and amphetamine-like drugs), cerebral vasodilators (e.g., papaverine), anabolic substances, and dihydroergotoxine mesylate (Hydergine). Hydergine, a dehydrogenated ergot alkaloid, in sublingual doses of 1–2 mg three times daily, has received some support as a means of improving cognitive function in the early phase of primary degenerative dementia (Ban, 1978a; Lehman & Ban, 1975; vonLoveren-Huyben et al., 1984; Yesavage et al., 1979).

Treatment of Alzheimer's dementia continues to be symptomatic-supportive, as already described in the general section of dementia. Proper patient management and family counseling are essential, and the only substantive services the physician can currently offer (Reisberg, 1982; Reisberg, Ferris, & Gershon, 1981).

The use of neuroleptics in the treatment of behavior symptoms in senile dementia of the Alzheimer type has recently been reevaluated. Earlier studies had shown that the target symptoms of agitation, hyperactivity, assaultiveness, irritability, and hallucinations are controlled by neuroleptics in 60% of patients (Rada & Kellner, 1976). However, several recent well designed placebo-controlled studies of neuroleptic medications in behaviorally disturbed dementia patients (mostly primary degenerative) have shown efficacy by global ratings in only one-third of the patients (Raskind & Risse, 1986).

Petrie et al. (1982) found only 32% of loxapine-treated patients (mean dose 22 mg/day) and 35% of haloperidol-treated patients (mean dose 4.6 mg/day) were globally rated as moderately or markedly improved. Target symptoms most responsive to the active drugs included suspiciousness, hallucinatory behavior, excitement, hostility, and uncooperativeness. Similarly, in a study by Barnes et al. (1982), thioridazine (mean dose 62.5 mg/day) and loxapine (mean dose 10.5 mg/day) produced marked or moderate global improvement in only one-third of the patients. Anxiety, excitement, and uncooperativeness were the most drug-responsive target symptoms. Steele et al. (1986) found both haloperidol (1, 2, and 5 mg/day) and thioridazine (25, 50, and 75 mg/

day) effective for managing behavioral symptoms in senile dementia of the Alzheimer type.

290.4x Multi-infarct Dementia

This is the second most common of the progressive dementias arising in the senium. It is characterized by a stepwise deteriorating course, focal neurological signs and symptoms, and evidence of significant cerebrovascular disease. Hypertension is a very common concomitant disorder. It is thought to be due to widespread multiple cerebral infarctions, secondary to cerebral arteriosclerosis. Risk factors predisposing to Multi-infarct Dementia include positive family history, hypertension, high serum cholesterol, serum triglyceride and lipoprotein profile associated with atherosclerosis, obesity, and smoking.

There is no known effective method for reversing or arresting the course of this dementia. Various drugs, such as anticoagulants, vasodilators (Hydergine, papaverine), and lipotropic enzymes have been proposed for altering the course of vascular disease (Cole & Braconnier, 1980; Lehman & Ban, 1975; Salzman, 1982). No reported controlled studies clearly prove the value of any of these agents. Recent reports on the potential usefulness of anti-platelet-agglutinating drugs, such as aspirin, in reducing the risk of infarction in patients with transient ischemic attacks may have some relevance in the treatment of Multi-infarct Dementia (Cole & Broconnier, 1980; Gaitz, Varner, & Overall, 1977; Hass, 1979). See also section on Multi-infarct Dementia with Delirium.

2. Psychoactive Substance-Induced Dementias

These are reversible dementias. The *DSM–III–R* lists on Axis I the following psychoactive substance-induced dementias of known etiology:

291.20 Dementia Associated with Alcoholism

Alcohol dementia is presumed to be caused by prolonged, heavy alcohol abuse. Its etiology is still controversial. It needs to be differentiated from subacute Wernicke-Korsakoff, traumatic, and hepatic encephalopathy. It is associated with greater than 10 years history of drinking and is nonprogressing if alcohol-free. There is evidence for cortical atrophy which may subside following prolonged abstinence (Francis & Franklin, 1987). There is no established specific treatment of this dementia. Abstinence from alcohol, use of thiamine, and good nutrition are recommended.

292.82 Other Psychoactive Substance Dementia

Numerous drugs have been reported to cause reversible dementia following long-term use or chronic intoxication. The most commonly implicated drugs include sedative-hypnotic-anxiolytics, other psychoactive drugs (e.g., lithium carbonate, cyclic antidepressants), beta blockers (e.g., propranolol), methyldopa (especially combined with haloperidol), clonidine (especially combined with fluphenazine), phenytoin, anticholinergic compounds, disulfiram, oral hypoglycemics, anti-inflammatory agents, cimetidine, digitalis, quinidine, L-dopa, diuretics, narcotics (Stoudemire & Thompson, 1981). Steroids can also produce dementia-like decline in cognitive functioning mimicking early Alzheimer's disease (Varney, Alexander, & MacIndoe, 1984). These dementias clear following discontinuation or reduction of medications.

3. Dementias Associated With Axis III Physical Disorders or Conditions

Most of the conditions listed in Table 1 may produce dementia coded as 294.10. They may be irreversible or reversible. Neurologic disorders associated with irreversible dementia include intracranial infections (e.g., encephalitis, Creutzfeldt-Jacob disease, neurosyphilis, HIV subacute encephalopathy in AIDS (Hoffman, 1984; Nichols & Ostrow, 1984), degenerative diseases (Pick's disease, Huntington's chorea, Parkinson's disease, progressive supranuclear palsy [Martin & Black, 1987]), vascular disorders (thrombotic and embolic strokes, Binswanger's disease, etc.), cerebral injury, intracranial space-occupying lesions (tumors, subdural hematoma, colloid cyst, etc.), and other CNS disorders (temporal lobe epilepsy, multiple sclerosis, etc.). Of particular interest are dementias caused by heavy metals and industrial poisons (lead, carbon monoxide), systemic lupus erythematosus, hypertensive encephalopathy, porphyria, Wilson's disease, hypoxia–anoxia, vitamin deficiencies (e.g., B1, B12), normal pressure hydrocephalus, carotid artery occlusal, temporal arteritis, cerebral abscess, Lyme disease, and other disorders. Early treatment of these last mentioned disorders may prevent the development of dementia or reverse it.

Eminently reversible dementias include endocrinopathies (hypothyroidism, Addison's disease), metabolic encephalopathies (diabetic acidosis, hepatic and renal failure, dialysis dementia), electrolyte/water imbalance, hypoxia due to cardiac or pulmonary disease, and Sjörgen's syndrome. It is beyond the scope of this book to review the specific treatments of these disorders.

Chapter 11

Syndromes Similar to Functional Disorders

11A: ORGANIC AMNESTIC SYNDROME

The Organic Amnestic Syndrome is characterized by a selective cognitive impairment in short- and long-term memory. The syndrome occurs in a state of clear awareness (differentiating it from Delirium) and without any significant loss of the remaining intellectual abilities (differentiating it from Dementia).

The syndrome results from bilateral lesions of specific diencephalic or medial temporal lobe structures (e.g., hippocampal formation, mammillary bodies, fornix, and structures in the floor and walls of the third ventricle). The lesions may be reversible or irreversible, depending on the etiology of the causative disorder.

Conditions associated with Amnestic Syndrome of either transient or persistent course include thiamine deficiency (e.g., Wernicke-Korsakoff syndrome), head trauma, carbon monoxide poisoning, subarachnoid hemorrhage, herpes simplex encephalitis, brain tumor, bilateral posterior cerebral arterial occlusion, and cerebral hypoxia. Conditions associated with transient amnestic syndrome include temporal lobe epilepsy, migraine attacks, chronic drug intoxication (e.g., barbiturates, bromides, isoniazid), and electroconvulsive therapy.

Treatment

Treatment is etiologic (when cause is known and treatable) and symptomatic. There is no symptomatic treatment to correct the cognitive deficit in memory. Physostigmine may improve the Amnestic Syndrome after herpes simplex encephalitis (Peters & Levin, 1977). Memory therapy (teaching the patient to use visual mnemonics) may be helpful to patients with preserved ability to retrieve visual images (Patten, 1972). Specialized rehabilitation programs in "cognitive retraining" are especially valuable, particularly for those with head trauma (Kwentus et al. 1985; Lezak, 1978).

Patient Management
Management approaches are similar to those described for demented patients. However, it should be noted that, compared with demented patients, amnestic patients suffer from a more circumscribed cognitive deficit, maintain relatively intact verbal capacities, and are less vulnerable to developing major psychiatric complications. Although institutionalized custodial care may be necessary for patients with more severe forms, most of these patients can be cared for at home or in a supervised, structured environment. Efforts at rehabilitation of patients with milder syndromes should always be part of the management plan.

SPECIFIC ORGANIC AMNESTIC DISORDERS
The *DSM-III-R* classifies organic amnestic disorders into substance-induced codes on Axis I, and others coded on Axis III.

1. Psychoactive Substance-Induced Amnestic Disorders
The most commonly implicated substances are alcohol and sedative-hypnotic drugs.

291.10 Alcohol Amnestic Disorder
This thiamine deficiency syndrome, also known as Wernicke-Korsakoff syndrome, is the most common amnestic syndrome. It is secondary to the nutritional deficit associated with chronic alcoholism. Brain lesions associated with thiamine deficiency include bilateral sclerosis of the mammillary bodies (Benson, 1978) and degenerative changes in the dorsal nucleus of the thalamus (Victor et al., 1971). In the majority of cases the onset is acute, presenting as a sequela of Wernicke's encephalopathy; a smaller number of patients experience an insidious onset without a preceding acute encephalopathic episode (Adams, 1983).

The reversibility of the Wernicke-Korsakoff syndrome depends on the promptness of instituting specific treatment with thiamine. Thiamine should initially be given parenterally in doses of 50 mg daily for about

sodium lactate; if there is no improvement, propranolol and lidocaine can be useful. Prolonged EKG monitoring is extremely important for diagnosing cardiac arrhythmias, and as a means of assessing severity or tricyclic intoxication. The latter correlates with the degree of widening of QRS complex and prolongation of QT interval (Goldfrank & Meliek, 1979; Granacher, Baldessarini, & Messner, 1976).

Section III
Psychoactive Substance Use Disorders

by

George U. Balis, M.D.

Chapter 13

Psychoactive Substance Use Disorders

This diagnostic class defines disorders with maladaptive behavioral changes associated with pathological use of psychoactive substances. They are distinguished into Psychoactive Substance Dependence and Psychoactive Substance Abuse.

Psychoactive Substance Dependence has been redefined by new criteria in *DSM-III-R*. The essential feature is a cluster of cognitive, behavioral, and physiologic symptoms that constitute a *dependence syndrome*, indicating that the person has impaired control of psychoactive substance use and continues its use in spite of adverse consequences. The diagnosis of the dependence syndrome requires at least three of nine characteristic symptoms of dependence, some of which have persisted for at least one month, or have occurred episodically over a longer period.

Psychoactive Substance Abuse is a residual category in which maladaptive patterns of psychoactive substance use have never met the criteria for dependence.

Personality disturbance and other psychopathology (e.g., depression, anxiety) are often present as associated features in substance use disorders. Complications resulting from Substance Abuse or Substance Dependence include substance-specific Organic Mental Syndromes, deterioration of physical health due to malnutrition and poor hygiene, and medical complications due to the effects of the substance (e.g., cirrhosis, peripheral neuropathy, acute pancreatitis associated with Alcohol Dependence) or due to the administration of the substance by contaminated needles (e.g., hepatitis, AIDS, vasculitis, septicemia in Opioid Dependence).

General Therapeutic Principles

The field is replete with treatment approaches, based on diverse theories and ideologies, with claims of therapeutic successes that generally lack objective substantiation. The following principles constitute general guidelines for a treatment and management plan.

1. There is no singular treatment modality that can claim high effectiveness for chemical dependence.
2. A combination of modalities is most likely to achieve a measure of therapeutic success.
3. The treatment modalities must be tailored to the individual, taking into consideration his or her specific problems, response to previous treatment attempts, and the resources available.
4. Different treatment and management approaches are administered by a great variety of professionals, nonprofessional practitioners, and lay groups. The physician plays a central role in the initial evaluation and medical diagnosis, management of physical/psychiatric complications, detoxification, and appropriate referral. In follow-up care, the general physician may apply some of the specific methods available, or may collaborate with other practitioners and various agencies involved in the treatment and rehabilitation of the patient.
5. A prerequisite for any treatment plan is the detoxification of the patient (see Treatment section on Withdrawal and Withdrawal Deliria).
6. The presence of associated psychopathology requires specialized psychiatric treatment, especially with regard to affective disorders and personality disorders (e.g., antisocial, borderline).
7. The socially dislocated individual (e.g., unemployed, homeless, legally entangled, or culturally alienated) requires social and vocational rehabilitation, with the goal of reintegrating him or her into the family, community, or work setting.

Treatment modalities currently include:

1. *Pharmacologic methods,* such as disulfiram for alcoholism, tricyclics for cocaine dependence, narcotic maintenance and narcotic antagonists for opioid dependence, and various psychotropic drugs for the short-term management of targeted symptoms of anxiety and depression following detoxification.
2. *Psychosocial methods,* including individual psychotherapy, group therapy, family therapy, conjoint therapy with spouse, contingency contracting behavior modification, aversive conditioning, and relaxation techniques.
3. *Sociotherapies,* such as various therapeutic communities (e.g., Synanon) and other residential programs.
4. *Self-support groups,* such as Alcoholics Anonymous, Al-Anon, Alateen, Narcotics Anonymous.
5. Various therapeutic, educational, occupational, inspirational, or humane programs, supported or sponsored by government agencies, industry, religious organizations (e.g., Salvation Army), and other community and volunteer agencies.

Common factors that appear to contribute to therapeutic success include:

1. Patience, perseverance, and commitment on the part of the therapist while working with a very difficult and frustrating patient who is suffering from a chronic and relapsing disorder. This should be laced with hopeful expectation, kindled by a caring and nurturing but firm attitude, tempered by a realistic appraisal of the patient's potential and limitations, and monitored for transference and countertransference problems.
2. Maintenance of abstinence during treatment and the setting of abstinence as the ultimate treatment goal.
3. A degree of coercion that ranges from subtle measures of substance control to commitment to a treatment facility. It may take the form of "contracts" that the patient is persuaded or forced to make with the therapist, spouse, or employer, in the face of crisis situations. Structured environments, disulfiram administered under supervision, or limit setting in therapy are other examples of therapeutic coercion.
4. Breaking through the defense of massive denial. A major effort during the initial phase of treatment is to help the patient to recognize and accept the problem.

5. Bolstering of the patient's wavering motivation to stay in treatment and remain abstinent.
6. Development of alternative coping styles to handle intense dysphoric affects, especially rage, guilt, anxiety, and depression; and boosting and maintenance of self-esteem.

SPECIFIC PSYCHOACTIVE SUBSTANCE USE DISORDERS

303.90   Alcohol Dependence
305.00   Alcohol Abuse

Detoxification is the first step of treatment of alcoholism. Detoxification and treatment of psychiatric complications of alcoholism (Organic Mental Syndromes) were discussed elsewhere (see Organic Mental Disorders in Chapter 11).

A comprehensive treatment approach is best. Several treatment modalities should be integrated into a treatment plan tailored to the individual and the resources available. The treatment plan may include psychotherapy, group therapy, family therapy, conjoint therapy, support groups, disulfiram, and short-term use of tranquilizers or antidepressants for targeted psychopathology (Gerard & Saenger, 1966). Alcoholics Anonymous is part of most successful programs. Al-Anon provides assistance to spouses of alcoholics through group support, while Alateen serves the needs of children of alcoholic parents. Referral of family members to these organizations should be part of the multiple treatment approach.

Halfway houses may be important treatment resources for patients with placement problems following detoxification and discharge. Vocational rehabilitation and social support agencies may be required for selected cases (Selzer, 1980). In most communities, there are comprehensive alcoholism treatment and rehabilitation programs, many of which are inpatient or residential.

The primary physician plays a crucial role in diagnosis and treatment. Dealing with the patient's denial must be early and decisive. Instruments such as the Michigan Alcoholism Screening Test (MAST) may serve as the first step in loosening the patient's defensive armor (Selzer et al., 1975). With acceptance of the problem and the establishment of a therapeutic alliance, the physician can proceed with negotiating a therapeutic contract (Brady et al., 1982). Long-term abstinence should be the goal. If this is not possible, a trial period of abstinence is an acceptable compromise. The contract should include means of deterrence and ways of monitoring compliance.

Disulfiram is effective in selected cases, especially when relapse is frequent. Baseline laboratory studies should be obtained and the patient fully instructed about the consequences of drinking within four days of ingestion of the drug. Disulfiram is then given, preferably at bedtime, in a loading dose of 500 mg daily for five to seven days, then continued on a daily maintenance dose of 250–500 mg.

A spouse or some other person should be involved in administering the disulfiram at least every three or four days to ensure compliance or the patient may visit the therapist or clinic every three or four days for observed ingestion. After the first month, a new contract is negotiated, with the patient assuming responsibility for control of his drinking (Goodwin, 1982). Disulfiram should not be allowed to take the place of AA or other support and therapeutic activities.

The psychotherapeutic approach is primarily supportive with many patients; the therapist plays an active and nurturing role while maintaining clear boundaries of separateness and setting firm limits that discourage acting out and enforce the abstinence rule (Wurmser, 1979). Family therapy can be crucial in the treatment of the alcoholic in view of the dysfunctional family systems associated with alcohol abuse (see Kaufman, 1985). Behavioral therapy techniques include relaxation, assertiveness training, self-control skills, aversive conditioning contingency contracting, broad spectrum behavioral treatments, and biofeedback (Emrick, 1974).

Benzodiazepines and small doses of low potency neuroleptics are recommended by some, but only for short-term use following detoxification, for control of anxiety (Rothstein, Cobble, & Sampson, 1976). Most clinicians and programs recommend a drug-free treatment regimen, especially during the first two-to-three weeks following withdrawal (Pattison, 1986).

In patients with a "double diagnosis," a concomitant primary psychiatric disorder (e.g., affective disorder) may play a causative role in the development of alcoholism or, conversely, alcoholism may be a major destabilizing factor. Psychiatric conditions most commonly associated with alcoholism include mood disorders (bipolar disorder, major depression, dysthymia), borderline personality, and antisocial personality. Psychiatric treatment, especially of mood disorders, should be provided concurrently with treatment of alcoholism.

304.0x   Opioid Dependence
305.5x   Opioid Abuse

Treatment programs for the opioid addict (mainly heroin) include methadone maintenance, maintenance with opioid antagonists, therapeutic communities, and various abstinence-oriented recovery programs. Most of these provide a combination of adjunctive approaches, such as group therapy, improvement of social skills, vocational training, job placement, and family counseling.

Methadone maintenance is the most common and most successful treatment for opioid dependence (Mirin & Meyer, 1978). It is offered in special clinics under close supervision and monitoring. Unlike heroin, methadone is long-acting (24 hours), and is orally effective. In usual doses (40–50 mg), it blocks opioid craving, while in much higher doses (100–120 mg) it blocks the euphoriant effects of opioids. The most significant effect for maintenance is the blocking of opioid craving (Goldstein & Judson, 1973).

In spite of some criticism, methadone maintenance is an effective and safe method that allows the opioid addict to change his lifestyle, stabilize his functioning, and reintegrate into the community. Treatment goals are reduction of illicit drug use, reduction of criminal activity, increased employability, increased self-esteem, and improvement in family and community functioning (Berger & Tinklenberg, 1979; Green, Meyer, & Shader, 1975; Kissin, Lowinson, & Millman, 1978).

According to FDA regulations, those eligible for methadone maintenance are individuals whose dependence on heroin has lasted longer than two years. It is indicated for addicts who have an extensive history of drug use and antisocial behavior and who have repeatedly failed to maintain abstinence. A typical methadone maintenance clinic provides daily administration of oral methadone, monitored with urinalysis, plus drug counseling and ancillary services, including in some instances individual psychotherapy and group therapy.

Several authors have noted that the methadone maintenance approach tends to reinforce the addict's identity as a member of the drug subculture and to perpetuate detrimental attitudes towards drug use. (Dole & Nyswander, 1976; Lennard, Epstein, & Rosenthal, 1972). Many patients continue to use other licit and illicit drugs (Ausabel, 1983), the most common being alcohol (O'Donnell, 1969).

Levo-alpha-acetyl-methadol (LAAM) is a long-acting congener of methadone, currently under investigation. It can be administered three times per week, thus affording greater treatment flexibility (Ling & Blaine, 1979).

Maintenance with opioid antagonists—cyclazocine, naloxone, naltrexone, and buprenorphine—is currently undergoing field trials as a new treatment approach. Its goal is to decondition the behaviors of opioid use and relapse (Whitlock & Evans, 1978), by blocking both the euphoria and the relief of conditioned abstinence symptoms of the former opioid abuser, including injection rituals (Resnick et al., 1979).

According to Greenstein and colleagues (1983), patients most likely to benefit from naltrexone therapy are socially stable (employed, married), self-motivated, and stabilized on low-dose methadone before detoxification from methadone and induction with naltrexone. Naltrexone is useful as an adjunct to other therapies.

Naltrexone induction therapy consists of the following steps:

1. Detoxification from heroin or methadone and establishment of a drug-free period of at least seven days post-heroin withdrawal, or 10 days post-methadone withdrawal.
2. Administration of naloxone challenge in the already abstinent patient (e.g., 0.8 mg subcutaneously or IV of naloxone should elicit no withdrawal).
3. An initial dose of 25 mg or 50 mg of naltrexone is administered, once the patient has been shown to be ready for naltrexone induction.
4. Maintenance naltrexone at 350 mg per week, given on a daily (50 mg/day), twice a week (150 mg on Mondays and 200 mg on Thursdays), or three times a week (100 mg on Mondays and Wednesdays and 150 mg Fridays) regimen.
5. Weekly screening of urine for drugs during the initial several months of treatment, as well as periodic physical examinations.

Therapeutic communities (e.g., Synanon, Odyssey House, Daytop, Phoenix House) are drug-free, full-time residential programs that attempt to rehabilitate and resocialize the drug addict through the use of a rigidly defined, experiential lifestyle that emphasizes group interaction, peer pressure, and self-government. Treatment in the typical therapeutic community lasts one to two years and generally focuses on extensive lifestyle change by means of forceful confrontation. Some have criticized this model as being excessively authoritarian (Ausabel, 1983). Others have noted that there is little methodologically vigorous evidence to substantiate the effectiveness of therapeutic communities (Romand, Forrest, & Kleber, 1975).

This model is thought to be most effective for the highly motivated individual who can complete the required program (Mirin & Meyer, 1978; Sells, 1979). In this regard, the model may not be very practical for many addicts. However, it may be a good choice for the addict with legal entanglements that have led to court referral (Klein & Miller, 1986). The current status and evolution of the therapeutic community was recently reviewed by DeLeon (1985).

Abstinence-oriented recovery models in various addiction treatment centers are based on the alcoholic recovery model (Alcoholic Anonymous) and the derivative self-help groups of Narcotics Anonymous (NA) and Chemical Dependency Anonymous (Bill, 1968).

A confrontational approach that aims to break the addict's denial of the seriousness and severity of his illness is essential to this model, which includes an educational approach as well. These are generally residential programs in which group therapy is the primary treatment modality and family participation is actively sought. Discharge planning provides for continued support and structure, required attendance of NA meetings, urine screens to monitor possible drug usage, aftercare groups, and individual or family therapy when needed. This approach is thought to be most useful for addicts in the early stages of addiction who are motivated for change (Klein & Miller, 1986).

Other outpatient, drug-free programs provide various resocialization experiences, such as group discussions, assistance with social and vocational problems, and recreational activities. Some are organized along the lines of a daytime therapeutic community (Sells, 1979).

Psychotherapy. In spite of the widespread opinion that individual psychotherapy is ineffective with opiate addicts, there are several studies which indicate that professional psychotherapy can provide addicts additional benefits when combined with standard drug counseling services in a methadone-maintenance program (Resnick et al., 1981). Short-term interpersonal psychotherapy was found to be effective by Klerman, Dimascio, & Weissman (1974) and by Weissman et al. (1976), but not by Rounsaville et al. (1983). Supportive-expressive and cognitive-behavioral psychotherapies have also been reported to be useful within the context of a methadone program (Woody et al., 1983). Several studies have provided some evidence that psychodynamic (Willett, 1973), cognitive-behavioral (Abrahms, 1979), and implosive (Hirt & Greenfield, 1979) group therapies may be helpful for this population. Psychotherapy is particularly indicated in patients with psychiatric symptoms. Opiate addicts show a high degree of psychopathology, and addiction itself may often be viewed as self-medication to avoid depression, anxiety, and other dysphoric symptoms (Khantzian, Mack, & Schatzberg, 1974; Wurmser, 1979). Opiate addicts may require more intensive treatment than is typically offered in methadone programs (McLellan et al., 1979). For more detailed information about the use of psychotherapy in opiate abuse, the reader is referred to a review by Woody et al. (1986).

Psychopharmacotherapy. This may be indicated in addicts presenting serious psychiatric symptoms, and especially depression. In a placebo-controlled study of the effect of doxepin on depressed opiate addicts in a methadone program, doxepin was shown to produce substantially greater reduction of depressive symptoms (Woody, O'Brien & Rickels, 1975). On the other hand, a more recent placebo-controlled study using imipramine (Kleber et al., 1983) found that the two treatment groups showed equal improvement. Outcome studies of long-term treatment and rehabilitation programs show that methadone maintenance and therapeutic communities are the most successful approaches (Sells, 1979; Simpson, 1981).

HIV. Finally, one should recognize the possibility of HIV and other infections of intravenous drug users who share needles, and the continuing spread of Acquired Immune Deficiency Syndrome (AIDS) among them. Recent statistics show that 25% of approximately one million people exposed to HIV are intravenous drug users and that 40% of IV drug users tested are HIV seropositive (Fry, 1986).

304.10 Sedative, Hypnotic, or Anxiolytic Dependence
305.40 Sedative, Hypnotic, or Anxiolytic Abuse
This disorder is often iatrogenically initiated and/or maintained. Indiscriminate or poorly supervised prescription of hypnotics and anxiolytic drugs, especially in the elderly, is not an uncommon practice. Younger people abuse these drugs for their intoxicating effect, to enhance the euphoria of opioids, or to counteract the stimulant effects of cocaine and amphetamine. Benzodiazepines are the most commonly abused drugs.

Detoxification is a prerequisite of any treatment approach (see Withdrawal section in Chapter 12). Following detoxification, the patient should be evaluated to rule out primary psychopathology (e.g., Major Depression) and be given appropriate treatment if necessary.

There are no controlled studies on the efficacy of psychotherapy on this type of drug abuse. The few older studies available indicate poor outcome (Anderson et al., 1972; Tennant, 1979). It has been suggested that psychotherapy and group therapy may be useful in the patient with psychiatric illness (Liskow, 1982).

304.50   Hallucinogen Dependence
305.30   Hallucinogen Abuse
304.30   Cannabis Dependence
305.20   Cannabis Abuse
304.50   Phencyclidine (PCP) or Similarly Acting
         Arylcyclohexylamine Dependence
305.90   Phencyclidine (PCP) or Similarly Acting
         Arylcyclohexylamine Abuse

These classes of substances, commonly referred to as "soft drugs," are discussed together because they share common aspects of epidemiology and pattern of use. They are often used within the context of a characteristic drug subculture (Balis, 1974).

Severity of the disorder varies according to the type of substance used, degree of dependence, and concomitant psychopathology. Polydrug abuse often involves alcohol. Underlying psychopathology is a common problem, especially with the polydrug abuser, and usually involves depression, personality disorders, or both. Treatment of the underlying disorder is necessary for the long-term rehabilitation.

Detoxification is a prerequisite to treatment (see respective sections). Individual and/or group therapy are recommended for most patients, although its efficacy has not been established (Berger & Tinklenberg, 1979). Referral to drug-free outpatient programs and utilization of community support agencies are important. Unfortunately, most patients are not well motivated; the majority drop out early in treatment (Anderson, O'Malley, & Lazare, 1972).

Residential programs, especially therapeutic communities with rigorously structured resocialization programs, provide the greatest chance for success, particularly for the highly motivated or legally constrained individual (Sells, 1979). Generally, the longer a person stays in treatment, the more favorable the outcome (Simpson, 1981).

304.20   Cocaine Dependence
305.60   Cocaine Abuse

There is no consensus regarding optimal treatment for cocaine use disorder. In general, cocaine treatment programs use the methods of

Alcoholics Anonymous, contingency contracting, and urine monitoring. Hospitalization is necessary for those with chronic free-base or IV use, with medical or psychiatric complications, and/or with concurrent dependence on other drugs (Gold & Dackis, 1984).

"Contingency contracting" (Anker & Crowley, 1982) is based on the patient's agreement to participate in a urine-monitoring program and to accept an aversive contingency in the event of either a cocaine-positive urine or failure to produce a urine sample. Current treatments emphasize psychological strategies (individual, group, family therapy) aimed at modifying addictive behaviors, with reported success rates of psychotherapy in the range of 40%–45% for experienced programs (Anker & Crowley, 1982; Kleber & Gawin, 1984).

Pharmacological approaches to Cocaine Abuse and Cocaine Dependence have recently been introduced, with some promising results especially for tricyclic antidepressants. Desipramine was shown in an open clinical trial by Gawin and Kleber (1984) to be effective as adjunct to psychotherapy in decreasing craving and promoting abstinence, regardless of whether an affective disorder was also present. On the other hand, lithium was effective only in cyclothymic subjects.

In a subsequent double-blind, placebo-controlled study by Gawin, Byck, and Kleber (1985), desipramine facilitated abstinence in both depressed and nondepressed cocaine abusers. Similar results were reported by Giannini et al. (1986). Several larger-scale studies are currently under way (Gawin, 1986). Most recently, amantadine, a dopamine agonist, was reported to attenuate cocaine abuse in methadone maintenance patients at doses of 200 mg b.i.d. (Handelsman, 1987).

304.40 Amphetamine or Similarly Acting Sympathomimetic Dependence
305.70 Amphetamine or Similarly Acting Sympathomimetic Abuse

There are no established treatment guidelines for this class of psychoactive drugs. Treatment approaches are similar to the psychosocial methods described in Cocaine Abuse and Cocaine Dependence (see section on Organic Delusional Disorders in Chapter 11).

304.60 Inhalant Dependence
305.90 Inhalant Abuse

Once abstinence is achieved (see section on Intoxication in Chapter 12), psychosocial interventions are necessary to prevent recurrence (Westermeyer, 1987). Concomitant psychopathology needs to be recognized and treated accordingly. Various psychotherapies, sociodrama, and vocational rehabilitation have been used to treat adolescent abusers (Stybel, 1977). Family intervention and the mobilization of community resources are particularly important in an effort to improve family functioning and socioeconomic setting (Nurcombe et al., 1970). Various social approaches have been used during "epidemics" of inhalant abuse (Westermeyer, 1987). The syndrome is very difficult to treat.

305.10   Nicotine Dependence

In contrast to other substance use disorders, Nicotine Dependence alone is not associated with impairment in social or occupational functioning. There are numerous treatment methods, reporting varying rates of success. Behavioral and psychotherapeutic techniques include aversive conditioning, desensitization, symptom substitution, covert desensitization, hypnotherapy, group therapy, relaxation training, supportive therapy, and education therapy (Katz, 1980; Orleans et al., 1981). No one technique has proved superior to others, and none has consistently shown long-term success rates in excess of 20% (Mann, Johnson, & Levine, 1986). Several educational programs are available for smokers interested in giving up the habit.

The best results are seen in programs that combine education with group therapy and support. In spite of reported high rates of success for some programs, the majority of smokers relapse. Pharmacological methods using lobeline sulfate (a nicotine agonist), sedatives, or psychostimulants have not been proven effective (Hunt & Bespalec, 1974; Jaffe & Jarvik, 1978; Jarvik et al., 1977).

Nicotine chewing gum has had some limited success (Hjalmarson, 1984; Schneider et al., 1983); however, a large follow-up study showed that nicotine vs. placebo gum vs. advice booklets produced no significant improvement over physician advice, as measured by abstinence rates at one year (Thoracic Society, 1983). There is some evidence that subjects with high nicotine tolerance are more apt to benefit from the use of nicotine gum (Fagerstrom, 1982; Hall et al., 1985; Jarvik & Schneider, 1984).

Propranolol has been reported to be effective (Farebrother et al., 1980). Similarly, clonidine, an alpha noradrenergic blocker, was recently reported to reduce craving for cigarettes (Glassman et al., 1984). Abrupt abstinence when motivation is high may be the best method for most patients (Jarvik et al., 1977).

304.90 Polysubstance Dependence

According to new *DSM-III-R* criteria, this classification is used when there has been repeated use, for at least six months, of three or more categories of psychoactive substances (not including nicotine and caffeine), but no single drug has predominated. During this period, the criteria have been met for dependence on psychoactive substances as a group, but not for any specific substance. Many polysubstance abusers follow an indiscriminate use of multiple drugs, while others follow a characteristic pattern of alternating psychostimulant drugs with sedative, hypnotic, or anxiolytic drugs or alcohol.

Polydrug abusers are more likely to show significant psychopathology than single-substance abusers. Treatment of the concomitant psychiatric disorder is of major significance. Detoxification of patients with mixed drug dependence was discussed in the Treatment section on Withdrawal and Withdrawal Deliria in Chapter 12. There are no established specific guidelines for the long-term treatment and rehabilitation of the polysubstance abuser. In general, treatment approaches are similar to those described in single substance dependence.

304.90 Psychoactive Substance Dependence Not Otherwise Specified
305.90 Psychoactive Substance Abuse Not Otherwise Specified

These are residual categories and need not be discussed separately. The reader is referred to the previous sections on Psychoactive Substance Use Disorders.

dopamine agonists such as bromocriptine may be used (Levinson & Simpson, 1987). Thioridazine has few extrapyramidal side effects.

The "rabbit syndrome," with rapid lip twitches, is a very unusual form of EPS, and should not be confused with tardive dyskinesia. It will usually respond to antiparkinsonian drugs.

Akathisia. This can easily be mistaken for anxiety or worsened psychosis. Restlessness is generally felt primarily in the legs, or as difficulty sitting still. It is a major source of discomfort, and should be treated. When found in the absence of pseudoparkinsonism, it may respond poorly to the usual antiparkinsonian, anticholinergic, or antihistaminic preparations, but often yields to benzodiazepines.

Acute dystonia. The majority of acute dystonic reactions occur within 24 hours of treatment, 90% by the third day (Sranek et al., 1986). They are painful and frightening, and often include torsion of the trunk and oculogyric crisis. They are more common in young males. Dystonic reactions (and other side effects as well) are often confused by the patient with "allergy." Patients who say they are "allergic" or "hypersensitive" to neuroleptics should be carefully questioned, since these effects are easily preventable in most cases and there are few alternatives for antipsychotic treatment.

Symptoms should be treated immediately with IM or IV medication. Benztropine, 1–2 mg IM, is usually sufficient, and about as rapidly acting as IV injection. Diphenhydramine (5–10 mg IV) or biperiden (2.5–5 mg IV) is effective as well. Oral antiparkinsonian drugs are preventive, and should be considered in young male patients both to prevent the dystonia and to enhance medication compliance.

Endocrine abnormalities. Many patients taking antipsychotics for long periods gain modest amounts of weight, and sometimes develop a fuller facies. Some of these effects, particularly in men, are probably related to increased prolactin levels, which in turn may lead to gynecomastia and/or lactation. Thioridazine is the neuroleptic most commonly associated with sexual dysfunction, including occasional impotence or retrograde ejaculation.

Increased seizure potential. This is frequently a concern in patients taking neuroleptic drugs, particularly the low-potency ones and promazine (rarely psychiatrically prescribed). In actual practice, seizures are very rare with proper medication dosage; however, patients with seizure disorders should be monitored until their stability is established. Patients who have taken overdoses or very large amounts of neuroleptics should be considered at risk.

ECG changes. The antipsychotic drug most likely to the alter the electrocardiogram is thioridazine (Mellaril). Serious arrhythmias are quite unusual, although a pretreatment ECG may be advisable when high doses are anticipated, or in patients at cardiac risk.

Ophthalmic effects. As already mentioned, anticholinergic effects frequently cause mild accommodation problems, particularly in the elderly. Thioridazine is associated with a well-known, serious retinopathy, almost always in doses above 800 mg per day. Small deposits of melanin in the lens or cornea, usually of no clinical significance, may appear with any of the phenothiazines, but are uncommon in other neuroleptics. Glaucoma is listed as a possible side effect for most of these drugs, primarily because of the anticholinergic effects and the theoretical vulnerability to narrow-angle disease. This potential has probably been considerably overstated in the literature (Reid, Blouin, & Schermer, 1976).

Photosensitivity and other skin reactions. Patients taking neuroleptics, particularly chlorpromazine, are often vulnerable to sunburn (which may exacerbate other temperature-regulation problems). Sunscreens are recommended. Inconvenient rashes, usually maculopapular, are common. Although these may represent real allergies or hypersensitivities, their importance should not be overplayed to the patient. An antihistamine (e.g., diphenhydramine) is usually effective, as is switching to another medication. If the rash continues, a clinical decision can be made as to whether treatment of the psychosis is more important than the dermatitis.

Liver toxicity. Because all of the neuroleptics are metabolized through the liver, most with some difficulty, it is important to establish baseline liver function levels and to be alert for clinical signs of hepatotoxicity. Mild elevations of liver enzymes are generally not contraindications for neuroleptic use. The phenothiazines are the most likely offenders, and should probably not be used in patients with significant cholestasis (Dossing & Andreasen, 1982; Simpson, Pi, & Sramek, 1984).

Agranulocytosis. Most cases of this rare adverse effect are related to chlorpromazine use, probably because of its high dose and low potency. Onset is usually within three months of the beginning of drug therapy, and most often involves high doses. Death is unusual, with recovery following standard supportive and antibiotic treatment for one to three weeks. Suddenness of onset precludes the effectiveness of serial monitoring of the white blood count; however, a baseline CBC is prudent. Patients frequently relapse if the phenothiazine is reinstituted; switching to a non-phenothiazine antipsychotic is recommended.

Tardive dystonia. This refers to the rare, rapid onset of abnormal movements similar to those seen in tardive dyskinesia, but more rapidly disabling, after even brief prescription of antipsychotic medication. Treatment is unclear. Very high doses of antiparkinsonism medications (e.g., 60 mg/day of trihexyphenidyl may be helpful for some patients. Stereotaxic surgery may be helpful in extreme cases (Goldman et al., 1985).

Neuroloptic-induced catatonia. This is an unusual syndrome which is difficult to differentiate from schizophrenic symptoms. A change of neuroleptic or prescription of amantadine is the accepted treatment.

Neuroleptics in pregnancy or during lactation. There is probably little risk in becoming pregnant while taking therapeutic doses of neuroleptics, although a few cases of congenital malformation possibly related to antipsychotic drugs have been reported. It is probably prudent to postpone drug treatment until the second trimester when clinically feasible; however, no definitive studies regarding the pros and cons of this practice have been done. Postnatal syndromes may be prevented by discontinuing medication at least 10 days before delivery. Since antipsychotic drugs enter breast milk, breast feeding should be discouraged.

Drug–drug interactions. As implied above, neuroleptics add to the sedative, CNS depressant, and anticholinergic effects of other drugs. They probably decrease blood levels of tricyclic antidepressants, and may decrease either the blood level or the anticonvulsant effect of phenytoin. The interactions of neuroleptics with cardiac preparations or pressor drugs must be considered for the individual agents involved. They probably increase the analgesic effects of pain relievers, including narcotics, either through drug interaction or through their own pain-dulling effects (see **Appendix A**).

Tardive Dyskinesia. Tardive dyskinesia (TD) is a serious adverse effect of all of the commonly prescribed antipsychotic medications. It is clear that not all patients—and perhaps not even most—will develop TD, even if taking neuroleptics for many years. Gardos and Casey (1984) describe the appearance of dyskinetic symptoms in 3%–4% of patients per year during the first five years of treatment, with older women perhaps being at greater risk. A very few patients develop lasting dyskinesia early in treatment.

Kane and Smith (1982) report an increasing incidence of TD, probably due primarily to recognition of the disorder. They suggest that about 15% of the patients chronically taking neuroleptics will develop the syndrome in some form; however, other studies have suggested higher rates. In any given year, roughly 4% of a neuroleptic-treated population of chronic patients develop dyskinetic symptoms (Kane et al., 1984).

The point-prevalence of persistent dyskinesia, based on a stable British cohort of schizophrenics, is about 12%. There is some indication that dyskinesia is only a transient feature for some patients, since at any particular time 41% of chronic schizophrenic patients in that cohort had some symptoms (Robinson & McCreadie, 1986).

Although there is little risk that the disorder will occur during brief hospitalization early in the course of drug therapy, successful prescribing of antipsychotic drugs often leads to a recommendation for months or years of similar treatment. The patient and his or her family should be given clear, accurate information about TD, its persistent nature, and the risks and benefits of accepting neuroleptic therapy. For the great majority of schizophrenic patients, the benefits of antipsychotic medication are significant. It should be carefully explained that TD almost always begins slowly, with symptoms that can be recognized early. At that point, a decision concerning treatment can be made, with the expectation that mild, early symptoms will probably remit if the medication is discontinued.

Dyskinetic symptoms frequently become temporarily worse after the medication is discontinued, and sometimes do not appear until that time. In the past, some authorities recommended masking these symptoms with increased neuroleptics; however, this practice is largely in disrepute.

Not all dyskinesia seen in psychiatric patients is related to antipsychotic medication. There is a natural rate of occurrence which may approach 5% in some populations without neuroleptics.

The cumulative dose of antipsychotic medication may be related to eventual development of dyskinesia; however, most recent evidence indicates that the total time the patient is on such drugs is probably the most important factor. "Drug holidays," changing neuroleptics, adding or not adding antiparkinsonism drugs, and so forth have not been consistently shown to prevent, or lessen the incidence of, this condition. Molindone may be less predisposing to tardive dyskinesia than other antipsychotic drugs; however, this has not been proved, and the therapeutic activity of molindone is probably less than that of the more established medications.

Symptoms. The patient should be examined for signs and symptoms of TD before and early in treatment, and at least every several months thereafter so long as the medication is prescribed.

Early symptoms of TD include mild, vermicular tongue movements, smacking of the lips, pressing the tongue against the cheeks, and chewing movements. Frequent examination for such movements should be carried out with the patient's mouth open and relaxed, while he or she is doing something distracting such as tapping the foot. Symptoms should be differentiated from other sources of mouth movements such as ill-fitting dentures; however, such movements should not be blamed on benign causes until TD has been ruled out. All dyskinetic movements can increase with various forms of stress and decrease when a patient is sedated. They generally disappear during sleep. Many patients deny that the movements are present, even while they are occurring.

The abnormal involuntary movement scale (AIMS) (see below) is a commonly used, rapid means of screening patients. It can be administered by trained, nonphysician personnel, but results should be reviewed by a psychiatrist or neurologist.

Abnormal Involuntary Movement Scale (AIMS)

- Have the patient sit in a hard chair without arms. Remove dental appliances, gum. Ask about dental or mouth problems.
- Observe and rate on the following scale: *0=no abnormality evident; 1=minimal abnormality; 2=mild; 3=moderate; 4=severe.*
- Record *individual and total ratings* for future comparisons.

____1. *Muscles of Facial Expression* (forehead, eyebrows, periorbit, cheeks; involuntary frowning, blinking, smiling, grimacing)
____2. *Perioral Muscles* (lip puckering, pouting, smacking)
____3. *Jaw* (biting, clenching, chewing, opening, lateral movements)
____4. *Tongue* (increased or vermiform movements)—Observe at rest in the mouth and when protruded; repeat.

____5. *Upper Extremities* (choreoathetoid movements)—Observe with hands hanging freely; omit tremors.

____6. *Lower Extremities* (choreathetoid movements, foot tapping, lateral knee movements)—Observe; may "activate" by distracting patient with finger exercises such as tapping fingers against thumb.

____7. *Neck, Trunk* (squirming, twisting, gyrating, rocking)—Observe sitting quietly, standing, standing with arms forward and palms down.

____8. *Overall Severity of Abnormal Movements*

____9. *Patient's Incapacity Due to Abnormal Movements*

___10. *Patient's Awareness of Abnormal Movements* (0=unaware . . . 4=aware and severely distressed by movements)

___11. *Current Dental Problems?* (0=no, 1=yes)

___12. *Usual Presence of Dental Appliances* (0=no, 1=yes)

Treatment of tardive dyskinesia is, at this point, entirely palliative and largely unsuccessful. There are a few patients who appear to respond to one of several different therapies (and a few whose symptoms remit spontaneously); however, none is broadly useful. Should symptoms be persistent or serious, neurological consultation is indicated.

Neuroleptic Malignant Syndrome. Neuroleptic malignant syndrome (NMS) is the most serious acute adverse effect of antipsychotic medications. Although rare, it is regularly reported in the literature, and has been seen at least a few times by most experienced clinicians. It affects all age groups, and, depending upon early recognition and treatment, may have a mortality of up to 20%. Significant mortality or morbidity is almost always associated with medical complications. Patients treated rapidly for their extrapyramidal symptoms, and promptly supported medically, are very likely to survive. Levinson and Simpson (1986) suggest naming the syndrome "EPS with fever" rather than "neuroleptic malignant syndrome."

At least 10%, and probably over 25%, of cases of NMS are probably related to nonneuroleptic causes (Levinson & Simpson, 1986). In some cases, severe EPS's interact with a medical condition to increase vulnerability. Perhaps only 20%–35% of apparent NMS appears in previously healthy patients.

Symptoms include rapid rise in body temperature, up to 105–107°F, severe EPS, muscle rigidity, elevated creatinine phosphokinase (CPK), and elevated white count. Although the condition appears to be related to basal ganglionic dysfunction, the actual mechanisms for the hyperthermia and rapidly altered sensorium are not entirely clear. Similar syndromes have occurred in patients on neuroleptics exposed to extreme heat or sunburn. The condition may recur in the same patient, making a change of medication and careful consideration of whether or not to continue neuroleptic therapy important concerns for the psychiatrist. Although molindone has been said to have a lowered risk of this and similar syndromes, cases of massive, life-threatening rhabdomyolysis with hyperthermia have been reported following its administration (Johnson et al., 1986).

Treatment of neuroleptic malignant syndrome. Treatment is fairly straightforward, and often successful. Neuroleptics should be discontinued and the patient immediately treated with bromocriptine, a dopamine agonist, orally 25–60 mg/day in divided doses (every three to four hours) (Rampertaat, 1986); amantadine orally 200–300 mg per day; or carbidopa/L-dopa orally up to 50/200 mg q.i.d. Bromocriptine is the most direct of these therapies. Muscle relaxant therapy such as dantrolene sodium 0.8–1.25 mg/kg IV or 50–200 mg/day orally (Lesser et al., 1986), or lorazepam 1.5–2.0 mg IV to start has also been effective. Support and cooling must accompany any of the above.

Other Drugs. *Lithium carbonate* is another nonneuroleptic drug sometimes used in schizophrenia. Although lithium may be a helpful adjunct to antipsychotic medication, and may address specific symptoms such as episodic violence or mood swings, it is not considered adequate treatment alone. Some patients with labile affective components of schizophrenic pathology, or patients who have been misdiagnosed as schizophrenic in the first place, may respond, however. "Schizophrenic" patients with affective or vacillating symptoms who have not responded well to neuroleptics should receive an adequate trial of lithium while continuing the antipsychotic regimen. The routine use of lithium to decrease aggressive or agitated behavior in schizophrenics is probably not warranted.

Judicious use of lithium and antipsychotic drugs together is not particularly dangerous, as was once thought. This is especially true if the lithium is added to a stable dose of an antipsychotic drug, and lithium levels are monitored appropriately. More detailed information may be found in Jefferson, Greist, and Ackerman (1983).

Naloxone has been carefully studied, but recent work indicates it is ineffective when prescribed alone for schizophrenia (Pickard Bartanian et al., 1982). The *benzodiazepines,* cited earlier for control of refractory acute psychosis, should not be considered adequate for ongoing antipsychotic treatment in schizophrenic disorders.

Pharmacologic milieu. As is the case for all other psychotropic medications, antipsychotic drugs should not be given in a therapeutic vacuum. The appropriate inpatient milieu for acute treatment has already been briefly outlined. In addition, the patient should understand the characteristics of his or her medication, its uses, its drawbacks, and its important place in the overall treatment plan.

Failure to continue needed medication is the single most common reason for relapse in discharged schizophrenic patients. The individual who understands his drug treatment, and who feels support from the psychiatrist, other psychotherapists, or family, is far more likely to feel he is an active participant in his treatment. This in turn may provide less need to manipulate the medication, less fear of its effects, a feeling of more control, greater optimism about one's destiny, and better understanding of the medication's role in rehabilitation.

Other Forms of Acute and Intermediate Antipsychotic Treatment. In addition to the pharmacologic approaches mentioned above, and expanded below for the treatment for refractory chronic patients, several other biologic, psychotherapeutic, special milieu, and dietary treatments have been tested during the past two decades.

Although *electroconvulsive therapy (ECT)* is useful for several types of acute schizophrenic episodes, most clinicians feel that pharmacologic treatment is preferable at all stages. It is unusual to see ECT used for routine treatment of schizophrenic patients in the United States or Canada (Salzman, 1980). If ECT is considered, one should adhere to the modern standards of practice described elsewhere in this text with regard to pretreatment protocol, consent, electrode placement, stimulus waveform, stimulus intensity, and number of treatments (Martin, 1986).

The possibility that dietary gluten may cause or affect schizophrenic symptoms has not been well proved in studies of *gluten-free diets* for schizophrenic patients. Most serious studies find little or no effect (Osborne et al., 1982; Potkin et al., 1981; Storms, Clopton, & Wright, 1982). Vlissides, Venulet, and Jenner (1986) carried out a 14-week double-blind trial of gluten-free diet in a psychiatric environment. They felt that most positive changes in their 27 subjects could be attributed to the attention they received; however, two patients did improve during the gluten-free period who relapsed when the gluten-containing diet was reintroduced.

Hemodialysis has been similarly disappointing in carefully controlled studies (Fogelson, Marder, & van Putten, 1980). *Luekotomy* is rarely used today except in the most intractable cases; however, at least one long-term follow-up suggests that carefully controlled psychosurgery may have been effective in the past in some patients, and probably led to less morbidity than is commonly assumed (Benson et al., 1981).

Outcome and Prognosis After Acute Treatment. Once the psychosis has remitted and reasonable psychosocial adaptation has occurred, the prognosis for many patients with schizophrenic, schizophreniform, and brief reactive psychoses is fair. In one study, over 70% of schizophrenic patients remained in remission at one-year follow-up (Rabiner, Wegner, & Kane, 1986). Premorbid factors such as inadequate social adjustment and longer duration of illness are correlated with poorer outcome. Three factors that appear to be very important to a good prognosis and that are under at least partial control of the psychiatrist are:

1. adequate intensity of hospital treatment
2. careful preparation for and transition to outpatient status
3. appropriate maintenance medication

The addition of paranoid psychosis to the schizophrenic syndrome complicates treatment and worsens the prognosis for most patients. The doctor–patient relationship is often strained, and the patient's paranoia interferes with his motivation for treatment compliance. Family and social adjustment tends to be poorer on average (Jorgensen, 1985). This may be because paranoid symptoms stand out in the community and are often more unsettling for others than are those of simple psychosis or psychotic withdrawal. It may also stem from our experience that paranoid delusions and hallucinations are more difficult to treat successfully. Review of the literature suggests that paranoid schizophrenics are commonly among those chosen for special "last resort" treatments for "intractable" or "treatment-resistant" patients (Brizer et al., 1985; Frances & Carpenter, 1983).

It is important to understand that although outward psychotic symptoms may rapidly remit during the first few weeks of hospital treatment, this does not necessarily indicate alleviation of all signs of the schizophrenic disorder itself, or of the depression and anxiety that accompany a psychotic break. One must focus treatment and follow-up on these aspects of care as well, and not merely upon the more visible psychotic signs (Szymanski, Simon, & Gutterman, 1983).

Work with the *families* of schizophrenic patients is important for preventing relapse, in part by helping the families develop the skills necessary to solve the many problems associated with schizophrenia, and in part by tempering some of the negative communication and relating among family members and the schizophrenic patient (Doane et al., 1986). Education about the illness, and particularly about maintenance medication, probably prevents or delays rehospitalization (Hogarty et al., 1986).

Supportive care in the *community*, including special clinics, social support networks, and short-term dynamic day hospital programs (defined separately from those for chronic patients) appear to increase quality of life and decrease use of both psychiatric and nonpsychiatric medical services (Glick et al, 1986; Schwartz et al, 1986; Vidalis & Baker, 1986).

One sometimes encounters efforts to incorporate meditative or "holistic" programs into the treatment milieu. Although patients may respond favorably during hospitalization, there is little information to indicate that such programs accelerate improvement, or that they have any positive effects on relapse rate, especially for chronic patients (Lukoff et al., 1986).

Suicide in Schizophrenia. The risk of completed suicide in schizophrenia is significant. The addition of an acute or subacute psychosis to the affective component sometimes seen in schizophrenic patients makes suicide attempts likely. At the same time, psychotic thinking makes attempts less predictable by clinicians or families, less organized, more impulsive, and sometimes more likely to be lethal.

Hopelessness concerning one's disease or social adaptation can be a contributing factor. Most schizophrenics are aware of their illness and of the fact that it may respond incompletely to medication. Withdrawal and ostracism by the community often lead to isolation. Suicide should be considered a possibility for all patients, and a probability for those who are particularly withdrawn or hopeless, or have a history of previous attempts. The "gesture"-like quality—or even bizarre nature—of previous attempts should not decrease one's caution about the seriousness of the patient's impulses. Schizophrenics may confuse self-directed and other-directed aggressive impulses, with a concomitant danger to others, particularly during acute psychosis. Drake, Gates, and Cotton (1986) feel that schizophrenics who have completed suicide may be distinct in many ways from the larger group of those who have attempted; however, they also advise caution because of the lower predictability of this group, compared to patients with affective disorders.

Chronic Schizophrenia

Outpatient Care. As noted above, the quality of the patient's transition from acute treatment to outpatient management has considerable bearing on adaptation and prognosis. Although patients differ, length and quality of remission are favorably affected by continuing medication in adequate doses and by consistent clinical follow-up.

Medication. Antipsychotic medication does not cure schizophrenia; it suppresses the symptoms. For patients whose diagnosis is Brief Reactive Psychosis (298.80) and who thus have specific stressors and time-limited psychoses, medication can usually be tapered and discontinued. Such tapering should be done with close monitoring by the psychiatrist, generally over several months, since tapering of the actual serum level does not closely follow decreases in dose, and the patient is in an environment quite different from that in which he or she received acute inpatient care (and often the same environment which precipitated the psychosis in the first place).

For those with Schizophreniform Disorder (295.40), the possibility of chronic schizophrenia is high. Drugs should be only cautiously tapered and discontinued, although such patients deserve at least one trial at being free of medication.

For patients with documented schizophrenic disorders or other psychoses which require continued antipsychotic medication, a decrease to maintenance dosage levels is recommended. This often decreases side effects and minimizes the total dose of neuroleptic received over the years during which the patient is likely to require such treatment. It is important, however, to wait until the patient's social situation has stabilized, with return to the family, establishment of office or clinic visits, return to work or school, and so forth, before changing the prescription significantly. Once this transition is complete, most patients can be maintained on as little as half or less of their acute treatment dosage.

The popularity of depot-injected medications for chronic schizophrenic patients is perhaps more related to marketing and pseudocommon sense than to any consistent recognition of its greater efficacy over other dosage forms and schedules. Several studies indicate that groups of patients receiving, for example, fluphenazine decanoate differ little from those taking oral fluphenazine at the same effective dose, although at least one large study (Babiker, 1987) indicates a slight— but statistically significant—lowering of rehospitalization rate among patients on the depot preparations. Interestingly, the highest rehospitalization rate in the Babiker study was found for patients taking both depot and oral antipsychotics.

Haloperidol decanoate has recently been introduced in the United States. It is said to have a slightly longer half-life than fluphenazine decanoate (up to four or five weeks), and is probably slightly less potent. There are few differences in side-effect profiles between fluphenazine and haloperidol, and any therapeutic differences may only be related to how often injections are given (and thus perhaps to bioavailability) (Wistedt, 1986). Other depot neuroleptics, such as zuclopenthixol decanoate (Kazi, 1986) and pipothiazine palmitate (Schmidt, 1986) are not yet available in the U.S. Some oral medications, such as pimozide, have long plasma half-lives and are effective when given less than once a day (McCreadie et al., 1982); however, most are not available in the United States.

The apparent advantages of depot medication are obvious: greater clinician control over patient compliance (and thus, apparently, over bioavailability), patient convenience in some cases, and assurance to the family and community (sometimes important in cases of committed or recently discharged violent patients) that drug treatment is continuing. Some of the *detriments* include the patient's feeling of lessened control over his or her care; misperceptions related to assault, penetration, or physical control by the caregiver; infantilization; limited choice of medication and side effect profile; and inability to rapidly discontinue the medication should serious side effects or adverse effects appear. No depot medication should be given without initial trials of nondepot preparations of the same active drug.

Medication compliance. Enlisting the active, positive participation of schizophrenic outpatients in their drug treatment draws upon the highest art of medicine. Many of the same issues mentioned under depot neuroleptic treatment must be frequently addressed. Each time the patient takes his or her medication, there is an opportunity for lowered self-image, frustration with the chronic illness, denial of need for the medication, rationalization for discontinuing it, and acting out within the therapeutic relationship.

If a previously stable patient begins to deteriorate or show early psychotic symptoms, the first thought should be related to whether or not he or she has taken his medication. Although one should not discourage patients' independence and autonomy, the use of family members, roommates, or even close friends as supports to help the patient make positive decisions about his or her treatment is recommended.

Deterioration does not always mean noncompliance, however. A number of factors may either decrease the bioavailability of antipsychotic medication or increase the patient's vulnerability to relapse. Some have to do with weakening of internal defenses. Intercurrent physical illness is a common source of deterioration. Even such simple things as cigarette smoking can significantly lower plasma neuroleptic concentrations (Jann et al., 1986).

The addition of other medications can either raise or lower (e.g., in the case of antiparkinsonian drugs) plasma levels through a variety of mechanisms. Assaying neuroleptic blood levels may help establish gross deficiencies for chronic outpatients or inpatients who have not responded after several weeks or whose response has markedly changed; however, such levels should not be used to titrate response (Faraone, Brown, & Laughren, 1987; Volavka & Cooper, 1987).

"Drug holidays"—which decrease total dose and perhaps the chance for tardive dyskinesia—have been suggested for many chronic patients. However, recent work by McMillan et al. (1986) indicates that even a two-day drug holiday may decrease serum levels of haloperidol by up to 40%. This probably does not correlate directly with CNS bioavailability; however, it may be a consideration in patients particularly prone to relapse or erratic drug response.

Intermittent medication. An alternative to simple maintenance of low dose antipsychotic medications for the chronic schizophrenic patient has been suggested by Marder and colleagues (1984), Carpenter and Heinrichs (1984), and others. Their approach recommends medication only when symptoms of psychosis or developing psychosis appear in the patient, reducing the neuroleptic dose considerably when the patient shows no psychotic symptoms. *This requires much closer monitoring* of chronic patients than is possible in many current social and treatment settings. This "intermittent" medication approach may also adversely affect treatment compliance for schizophrenic patients in general, since it may support denial and rationalizations for stopping medication when not recommended.

Chronic schizophrenic patients, particularly those refractory to traditional medication regimens, often deserve carefully monitored *pharmacological adjuncts* to their neuroleptic medication in order to reverse firmly entrenched symptoms or maximize improvement. In some cases, simply switching to a different class of antipsychotic may be helpful (sometimes because of enhanced bioavailability or selective receptor blockade): for example, changing from long-chain phenothiazines to mesoridazine or thioridazine (Vital-Herne et al., 1986).

Pharmacological adjuncts to continuing antipsychotic medication include the benzopyrones (Casley-Smith et al., 1986), reserpine (Berlant, 1986), thyrotropin-releasing hormone (TRH), and vasopressin (Branbilla et al., 1986). The benzopyrones were associated with statistically significant improvement in 16 clinic schizophrenic subjects treated for three months. The effect appeared to begin at about two weeks.

Reserpine, which has been associated with iatrogenic depression when prescribed for hypertension, has recently been associated with a moderate to dramatic response rate in 50% of 36 chronically disabled psychotic patients (Berlant, 1986). TRH (in doses of 600 micrograms IV every other day) and vasopressin (EDAVP) (4 micrograms IV every other day) were associated with improvement particularly in negative symptoms and memory of 23 chronic, undifferentiated schizophrenics who had responded poorly to neuroleptics alone. TRH treatment produced transient mild hyperthyroidism after about two weeks of treatment (Branbilla et al., 1986).

The "negative" symptoms of schizophrenia tend to be more troublesome than acute hallucinations or delusions. The addition of monoamine oxidase inhibitors (MAOIs) to neuroleptic therapy has been helpful in some treatment-resistant patients, and is considered safe when carefully monitored by the clinician (Bucci, 1987). Pipothiazine is a neuroleptic which may be particularly helpful for negative and affective symptoms (Schmidt, 1986).

Community Resources for the Chronic Patient. Available data indicate that some 75% of the primarily schizophrenic, chronically mentally ill lead lives with inadequate social adjustment. Talbott (1982) feels that no more than 25% of these patients get acceptable aftercare in addition to medication. He reports that housing is the most critical need for these patients, and reminds us that the incidence of medical illness for this group is roughly three times that of the general population.

Continuity of care is reasonably available to some patient groups, particularly in public sector settings such as the Veterans Administration hospital system. Mere availability of programs of social skills, education, and modification of disturbing behaviors does not, however, guarantee that patients will know about them, that they will be available in a practical sense (e.g., that appropriate transportation will be available), or that patients or families will want to take advantage of them. In spite of evidence that very active community support programs may reduce rehospitalization rates by up to 80% over rates seen with medication-oriented aftercare, both public and private payers, such as insurance companies or health maintenance organizations (HMOs), rarely fund such care.

Self-help groups can be enormously useful for many patients. There are now organized groups such as Recovery, Inc., the National Alliance for the Mentally Ill, and smaller groups devoted to particular disorders (such as the Depression and Manic–Depressive Association) in most large cities. Clinicians, particularly physicians, sometimes complain that information disseminated by self-help groups is inaccurate, or that patients' association with such groups can promote treatment noncompliance. One should learn about the quality and availability of self-help groups in one's own community, and then should offer lay-oriented information and guidance.

Chronic Hospital or Residential Settings. Return to the community is not possible for all chronic schizophrenic patients. Some maintenance treatment programs must take place in residential settings such as mental hospitals or nursing homes. Adequate psychiatric and other medical care, along with appropriate housing, educational and vocational opportunity, social skills training and recreation, should be provided. The concept of milieu or community should be at its best in the chronic-care institution. Nursing-home-like facilities tend to be inadequate substitutes, but are necessary in many locales.

The inpatient therapeutic setting should provide goals that are modest rather than far-reaching, and gentle support rather than intense or overstimulating settings. Unless the facility and its staff are equipped to deal with the regression and patient frustration that arise when treatment goals are overwhelming, the milieu should focus upon long-term adjustment as well as symptom removal (Drake & Sederer, 1986a).

There are a few hospitals in which long-term care is also considered acute treatment. In such highly specialized settings, the patient receives appropriate pharmacological treatment, becomes involved in an intensive attempt to bolster needed defenses and, to some extent, restructures portions of the personality that can become foundations for more effective adaptation.

These approaches are generally psychoanalytically oriented, although they may also follow learning theory approaches, and require great investments of energy, time, and money on the part of the patient and the clinical staff. For selected patients, the results are often better than those expected for those receiving only brief hospitalization and community follow-up or ordinary institutional care. The expertise and resources necessary for this work are unavailable to most patients, however, and may not be appropriate for many, provided good brief hospitalization and biopsychosocial follow-up are available.

A final long-term treatment modality, which should be mentioned but has not proved itself, is the community residential facility which encourages patients to view their psychotic episodes as useful life events or learning experiences. Such programs, sometimes supported by psychiatrists, appear to work well for a small subset of patients, perhaps those who would have done well in any event (and may not, in retrospect, have been schizophrenic). The environment is extremely accepting, usually homelike, with great support and encouragement to experience psychotic symptoms without anxiety, as a sort of temporary phase of life.

There is a difference between the above, global approach to schizophrenic illness and supportive psychotherapy for patients who are experiencing frightening delusions or hallucinations. Alleviating the anxiety associated with psychosis is an important, kind thing for the clinician to do. It may be done psychotherapeutically with support and reassurance, pharmacologically, or, for some patients, with insight. (See also the section on Psychotherapy of Schizophrenia, p. 194.)

Prognosis. Ratey, Sands, and O'Driscoll (1986) have recently written an interesting paper on the phenomenology of recovery for these patients. Outcome studies which in the past indicated that about one-third of schizophrenic patients returned to near-baseline emotional and social functioning after their first psychotic episode, with another third faring quite poorly, were often based on diagnostic criteria which today are felt to be overly broad, and probably included many patients with brief reactive psychoses.

Thirty-eight-year follow-up of a rural British cohort indicated complete recovery for almost 30%, with permanent disability in about 35% (Watts, 1985). An important German study indicated that about 22% of schizophrenics demonstrated complete recovery, with 56% "socially recovered." About two-thirds of the patients regained their level of premorbid functioning after acute episodes. This study separated several subtypes of psychosis, including schizoaffective, and found the schizophrenic population to contain several types. About one-quarter had a very unfavorable prognosis (Gross & Huber, 1986).

A complete discussion of social outcome and utilization of medical services in a European cohort is found in Biehl and colleagues (1986). A Japanese study, which may not represent the behavior of similar patients in western cultures, nonetheless gives international corroboration to the general medical finding that earlier onset, longer duration of prodromal signs, and longer time periods between onset and first clinical presentation, predict poor psychosocial outcome (Inoue, Nakajima, & Kato, 1986).

Paranoid schizophrenics appear to respond better to acute treatment with the phenothiazines or other neuroleptics than nonparanoid schizophrenics. Individual and group psychotherapy, as well as milieu therapy, are generally supported in the literature; however, they have not been systematically evaluated. There is a greater likelihood of relapse for patients with paranoid symptoms, when compared with nonparanoid schizophrenics, when remission occurs without chronic deterioration. In general, paranoid patients tend to have better recovery of social function, in spite of the poor prognosis for full remission of symptoms. Premorbid adjustment is an important predictor of remission (Ritzler, 1981).

There is no doubt that the attitudes of patient and family contribute to the substrate of schizophrenic illness and help determine the level of recovery for individual patients. A combination of education and support is useful. Community supports, including day hospitals, appear to be beneficial for many patients, not just those who have few other social resources (Vidalis & Baker, 1986).

Many clinicians and social scientists feel that the biologic and social resources available for helping the chronic schizophrenic are, at least for the time being, largely exhausted. Gralnick (1986), for example, points to increasingly brief hospital stays (largely for financial reasons) focused on medication as the primary form of treatment, and burgeoning numbers of severely disabled, socially bereft patients. Many community alternatives need not be nearly so expensive as "back ward" care for the seriously disabled chronic patient and may be clinically preferable (Dickey et al., 1986).

Psychotherapy of Schizophrenia

Psychotherapy as a Primary Treatment. There are a number of psychotherapists and psychoanalysts who treat subacute schizophrenic illness with psychodynamic psychotherapy (with or without medication). This approach cannot be recommended to all clinicians, since the psychotherapy of severe emotional disorders, particularly those involving thought disorder, should be viewed as a subspecialty requiring particular training, skill, and experience. A number of principles for the psychotherapy of schizophrenia have been outlined by Arieti (1980):

1. The therapist should attempt to cause little or no anxiety early in treatment, and should try to diminish anxiety which is already present.
2. The therapist should not wish merely to return the patient to his or her premorbid condition.
3. The therapist must be able to provide and tolerate a delicate balance within the patient, sometimes for several years, before independence from therapy can be achieved.
4. Treatment must be seen as a way in which the patient proceeds toward gradual acceptance of the self.

The first two of these are quite different from psychotherapy of the healthier or "neurotic" patient. This treatment approach is an arduous task for all concerned; both therapist and patient must understand the requirements of time and energy involved.

Psychotherapy as Adjunct to Medication and Milieu. Carpenter, Heinrichs, and Hanlon (1986) have recently reviewed several approaches to interpersonal treatment of schizophrenia. D'Angelo and Wolowitz (1986) summarize the generally held suggestion of two distinct styles of recovery from schizophrenic episodes: *integration* and *sealing over*. It may be that patients able to integrate psychotic experiences have less primitive characters or defensive systems than those who deny or repress ("seal over") such experiences. On the other hand, the "integrators" may represent a separate diagnostic group.

The potential adverse effects of intensive milieu or psychotherapeutic treatment have been described in this chapter and in additional work by Drake and Sederer (1986b). McGlashan (1983) provides another review of intensive individual psychotherapeutic treatments.

The presence of a family into which the patient can be reintegrated is important; many therapists emphasize the family as a major part of restoration of the patient. Although the therapist may recognize serious pathology in the family, which may have victimized or scapegoated the patient, focusing intently on these problems and refusing to support the family until they are solved may interfere with the patient's reintegration.

Group psychotherapy with schizophrenics should be practical, be oriented toward support and social skills, and promote the beginning or sustaining of interpersonal relationships. Groups whose primary goal is facilitation of insight tend to be unsuccessful in ordinary inpatient or outpatient treatment settings (Mosher & Keith, 1979). Johnson et al. (1986) discussed the "pairing group." Groups that focus on day-to-day issues of community within structured inpatient, day hospital, or outpatient settings appear to be very helpful and gratifying for patients in these environments.

Tardive Dyskinesia and the Chronic Schizophrenic Patient

In a number of patients, symptoms of tardive dyskinesia will appear after several years of neuroleptic medication. In some others, symptoms may appear when antipsychotic drugs are discontinued, and may be confused with the more benign "withdrawal–emergent dyskinesia."

Since there is at present no treatment approach which is accepted as effective, the prospect of tardive dyskinesia is truly upsetting for patients and clinicians alike. The benefits of appropriate neuroleptic treatment for chronic schizophrenic patients generally outweigh the risks of developing a serious movement disorder, however. This is especially true when one considers the tremendous morbidity of schizophrenic illness, our increasing diagnostic accuracy, the probability that medications will be found in the future that either do not induce tardive dyskinesia or can be used to treat it effectively, and the fact that the dyskinesias almost always develop slowly and are often not permanent in the early stages. There is time for complex treatment decisions when and if symptoms first appear. (See pp. 180–181 for a more complete discussion of recognition and management.)

When stopping medication after several years of neuroleptic therapy, one may wish to carefully taper the antipsychotic to allow (in theory) dopamine receptors to become less hypersensitive. This does not always protect the patient against the exacerbation of dyskinetic symptoms, however. In those cases in which the physician decides that a neuroleptic should be used to mask dyskinetic effects—cases that should be quite rare—Branchy, Branchy, and Richardson (1981) report that a dose of approximately one-eighth of the maintenance dose is generally sufficient for the masking purpose.

295.6x   Schizophrenia, Residual

The treatment of residual schizophrenia largely parallels that of maintenance treatment for the other forms of schizophrenia. Because of the prominence of social and "negative" symptoms rather than acute psychosis, one may wish particularly to focus on those sections of the foregoing chapter that address interpersonal and social functioning, and pharmacologic attempts to restore appropriate affect and demeanor.

Chapter 15

Delusional (Paranoid) Disorder

297.10   Delusional (Paranoid) Disorder
        Erotomanic Type
        Grandiose Type
        Jealous Type
        Persecutory Type
        Somatic Type
        Unspecified Type

Acute Treatment. Acute psychotic presentation of Delusional (Paranoid) Disorder, differentiated from schizophreniform illness, affective illness, organically induced paranoia, or paranoid personality, is unusual. The literature reflects a number of case reports and studies of paranoid disorders which eventually show themselves to be related to schizophrenia, or which follow a deteriorating course.

These are not the topic of this brief chapter, but are best treated with careful medical and psychiatric evaluation, antipsychotic medication, and follow-up similar to that of Brief Reactive Psychosis or Schizophreniform Disorder. They are sometimes confused with paraphrenia, a late-onset form of schizophrenia (Bridge & Wyatt, 1980; Jorgensen & Munk-Jorgensen, 1985; Varner & Gaitz, 1982). Some atypical paranoid psychoses respond to antidepressant pharmacotherapy, with or without neuroleptics (Akiskal et al., 1983).

Because of the generally normal vocational functioning but possibly deteriorating social or marital functioning in Paranoid (Delusional) Disorder, and the absence of hallucinations or evidence of acute psychosis or organic disorder, the initial setting for evaluation or treatment is likely to be the psychiatrist's office (sometimes a forensic psychiatrist, for persons whose delusions have begun to impinge upon the rights of others). If the presentation is such that others appear to be in danger (e.g., the patient seems about to take action based upon delusions of persecution or jealousy), then physical management such as hospitalization may be indicated. For those patients who have evidenced dangerousness, a secure facility or referral to a law enforcement agency may be the best course.

A number of physical and environmental influences may precipitate paranoid delusions. Deafness, for example, particularly in the elderly, may be a treatable cause of the delusions and may cause one to change the diagnosis. Persons recently separated from distant cultures, particularly eastern cultures, may respond either to understanding or, in some cases, to return to that culture (Waynik, 1985). Much of the literature focuses upon patients who are elderly or medically ill; these cases are most often related to dementia, other organic causes, or environmental deprivation.

A few studies indicate that pure paranoia is not well treated with antipsychotic medications or ECT (Astrup, 1984). Most patients are reluctant to take neuroleptics, although they are effective in some cases.

The author has seen several cases of paranoia, with and without delusions, related to vitamin absorption syndromes such as pernicious anemia (Zucker et al., 1981). Even when no anemia can be found, a trial of intramuscular vitamin B-12 is inexpensive and easily accepted by the patient.

In general, the longer the symptoms have been present, the more refractory they are to simple treatment such as explanation, education, or medication. Some culturally induced syndromes may respond to relocation, even if they have taken months to come to clinical attention, however.

Psychotherapy, when accepted, tends to be the treatment of choice, and should be begun in such a way that the patient is likely to see some benefit from it and some support from the therapist. The therapist should be alert for the appearance of other sources for the paranoia and should be qualified to evaluate them as they arise. There is some evidence that systematic desensitization may be effective in reducing delusional behavior; however, generalization to other parts of the patient's life is limited (Ritzler, 1981).

The patient is often quite uncomfortable, particularly in situations of persecutory, somatic, or even erotomanic delusions. A good therapeutic relationship may at least prevent the patient from taking action which might be destructive to himself or others, and may help with family relationships. Counseling for family members is usually welcomed.

Chapter 16

Psychotic Disorders Not Elsewhere Classified

298.80 Brief Reactive Psychosis

Remembering the caveat *primum no nocere*, it is often prudent to allow the acutely psychotic patient about whom little is known to go without neuroleptic or thymoleptic medication for a few hours (or even a few days), provided he or she is not extremely uncomfortable or threatening to others. Placing the patient in a protected environment, away from possible psychosocial or chemical sources of his or her psychosis (e.g., great stress, drug or chemical exposures) will often allow the symptoms to clear, sometimes completely. Psychoses related to, for example, unusual reactions to incarceration (e.g., the dissociative "Ganser syndrome"), sleep deprivation, chemical exposure in the workplace, surreptitious drug abuse, intentional or accidental poisoning, and the like should clear with simple medical support. Neuroleptics, with their long durations of action and many side effects, can significantly cloud the diagnostic picture and have been responsible for more than a few patients' appearing to be psychotic long after the initial source of the symptoms was gone.

When early, acute restraint or sedation is necessary to protect the patient or to make him comfortable, short-acting barbiturates or short-acting benzodiazepine anxiolytics are usually sufficient. Humane physical restraint or seclusion may be preferable to medicating a patient whose history is unclear during the first few hours of treatment.

In many cases, of course, antipsychotic drugs will be needed. They should be prescribed using the guidelines for emergency and acute treatment in Chapter 14.

After the acute psychosis has abated, more complete recovery may take considerable time. The person's emotional vulnerability to psychosis, presence of precipitating factors in the home or work environment, history of illness and prescribed or nonprescribed drugs, and so forth must all be evaluated. Treatment should continue, on an open psychiatric unit if possible, until the patient is ready to return to the outpatient setting. The transition from the hospital should be certain to include at least some outpatient contact which focuses on support and reorganization, and efforts to prevent future problems.

295.40 Schizophreniform Disorder

Since this disorder meets virtually all criteria for schizophrenia except that of symptom duration, treatment of the acute, early, and even some maintenance stages are essentially as described in the chapter on schizophrenia (Chapter 14). The possibility that the patient has schizophrenia should be carefully considered, although the diagnostic label should be avoided until it is clear. The symptoms of thought disorder should be carefully monitored after discharge from acute hospitalization. As with brief reactive psychosis, one should carefully consider whether any continuing symptoms are related to the illness, or to medication that is being prescribed.

Although schizophrenia may be diagnosed later, a number of patients with Schizophreniform Disorder will remain free of psychosis on little or no medication. The clinician should cautiously decrease maintenance medication and attempt to discontinue drugs in those patients whose symptoms are in good remission. Frequent monitoring with brief office visits and/or family contact for a few months after the psychosis has abated is good practice, and is usually appreciated by patients and their families.

295.70 Schizoaffective Disorder

Because of the poorly defined, "residual" nature of the *DSM-III-R* category, Schizoaffective Disorder, no specific treatment is recommended. Primary treatment should be provided for the particular clinical form taken by the disorder. That is, if a patient exhibits schizophreniform symptoms, treatments similar to those recommended for the schizophrenias (Chapter 14) should be one's first choice. Conversely, if the symptoms of thought disorder seem secondary to marked affective characteristics, such as depression, hypomania, or lability of mood, then lithium and/or antidepressant regimens should be considered in much the same way as is described in the chapter on Mood Disorders (Chapter 17).

There is no reason not to consider a combination of neuroleptic and thymoleptic (antidepressant) medication. The first—neuroleptic or thymoleptic—should be stabilized before the second is added. The patient may respond favorably and obviate any need for additional drugs. Fixed-dose combination preparations should be avoided. As previously stressed, the nonpharmacological components in treatment of both schizophrenic and affective disorders should receive careful consideration in the overall care of the patient.

Among the types listed in the *DSM-III-R* (bipolar or depressive), treatment of the depressive patient without clear psychotic or manic symptoms, but with symptoms similar to the "negative" symptoms of schizophrenia, is probably more difficult than treatment of other types. It should be remembered that the antidepressants of choice are likely to take at least three or four weeks to show their effect, and that the patient's response (or apparent response) may be delayed by schizophreniform symptoms. As is the case with other severely depressed or suicidal patients, serious suicide risk, morbid withdrawal, or manic or catatonic agitation unresponsive to medication are all indications for electroconvulsive therapy. The course of this disorder is not well known, largely because of its diagnostic vagaries and the probability that the patient later will be shown to have either a thought disorder or an affective disorder. There is some evidence that maintenance antipsychotic medication should not be used for as long a period as for schizophrenic patients.

Finally, one should note that dysphoria is a common symptom in schizophrenia. Drug-induced or post-psychotic depressions are common. These and akinetic effects of antipsychotic drugs may be mistaken for schizoaffective withdrawal and psychomotor retardation.

297.30   Induced Psychotic Disorder

In Induced Psychotic Disorder, or similar disorders with other names (shared paranoid disorder, *folie à deux*), many clinicians recommend separation of the persons involved. The secondary patient, whose delusions began after those of the person with a primary disorder, may particularly respond to such separation. This is especially true if the patient is the child of a psychotic "primary." Hospitalization should be considered in order to provide a supportive environment in which the patient's loss can be resolved and more productive defenses strengthened. Medication may be necessary either for psychosis or for the affective symptoms that may develop.

Confrontation alone, sometimes attempted when the "secondary" patient merely appears to be immature, should be avoided unless a more complete therapeutic context can be offered. Although the patient may not wish vigorous treatment, and may avoid it, the clinician should remember that sooner or later the patient will separate from the "primary," perhaps, for example, through the death of a psychotic parent. Preparation for this event, and support when it occurs, may prevent further decompensation.

298.90 Psychotic Disorder Not Otherwise Specified (Atypical Psychosis)

Atypical psychoses should by and large be treated symptomatically, using the principles outlined for more specific disorders elsewhere in this book. Early treatment should always include careful evaluation for organic, environmental, or other psychosocial causes of the psychosis that might lead one toward or away from certain interventions.

When rapid control of acute agitation is imperative for complete evaluation, in order to implement necessary medical treatment, or to prevent damage to the patient or others, short-acting barbiturates may be useful without masking important symptoms. Low doses of haloperidol or other potent antipsychotics are safe and may be effective. Neither should be given before evaluating the medical status of the patient.

Chapter 17

Mood Disorders

17A BIPOLAR DISORDERS

(*Note:* See Chapter 14 for more detailed descriptions of inpatient setting and milieu. See p. 219 for discussion of antidepressants.)

296.4x Bipolar Disorder, Manic
296.6x Bipolar Disorder, Mixed, Manic Phase

Emergency Treatment. Acute mania should be considered a medical emergency. It can result in severe physical decompensation or death if not treated properly. Although the *DSM-III-R* allows for mild or moderate manic episodes, the paragraphs below refer to patients who are in a state of marked physical and mental stimulation, who often have not slept for at least 24 hours, and whose exertion may exceed safe limits.

The first goal of treatment is rapid, safe calming of the patient within a medically supervised setting. Sedation with antipsychotic medication,* IM if necessary initially, is one treatment choice. Some clinicians prefer the "rapid neuroleptization schedule" described in Chapter 14. Others prefer more sedative drugs, such as chlorpromazine. In either case, one should expect the patient to require larger amounts than similar patients with other kinds of neuroleptic-responsive psychosis (e.g., schizophreniform psychosis), and should plan to use the neuroleptic for only a short time. Monitoring of medical status, particularly

---

*The reader is referred to **Appendix B** for generic and trade names of medications.

blood pressure, is necessary. Medication side effects such as dystonia, tremor, or anticholinergic effects may appear and should be promptly treated.

The use of short-acting barbiturates is highly recommended for simple sedation of patients with acute psychotic agitation. These have the advantage of controlling the physical dangers without most neuroleptic side effects, and mask fewer symptoms of psychiatric or medical illness. ECT has been recommended for life-threatening mania, unless or until pharmacologic regimens can take effect. The course of ECT should be routine, rather than only two or three treatments to control immediate symptoms.

Post-Emergency Acute Treatment. Most patients present for treatment with moderate mania or hypomania. The clinician should determine whether the patient has previously responded to a particular drug regimen which has been discontinued, and which could be reinstituted with probable success. The patient should be hospitalized during this time, for continuing evaluation, monitoring of response, assuring compliance with treatment, and psychosocial preparation to return to the community.

If the patient is unfamiliar to the clinician or has just received emergency treatment for mania, the pharmacologic aspects of the treatment plan should include starting oral lithium carbonate, with initial control of symptoms using neuroleptic medication. One should expect the lithium to take effect within one to one-and-a-half weeks of reaching an appropriate serum level.

Pre-lithium workup. Healthy patients under 40 years of age can safely be started on lithium after a routine medical history; physical exam; and laboratory determination of normal CBC, electrolytes, kidney function, and thyroid function. Patients over 40 (or those with histories of heart disease) should receive an electrocardiogram. If there is any suspicion of compromised renal function, then creatinine clearance, urine concentrating ability, and urine output should be evaluated. After therapeutic levels have been stable for a few weeks, the blood chemistries should be repeated.

Although many psychiatrists occasionally start lithium treatment on an outpatient basis, inpatient treatment is prudent, particularly for patients whose psychiatric problems make compliance difficult, patients who might take an overdose of the medication, or those requiring close medical monitoring. Most patients discussed in this section will be hospitalized for 10 to 30 days.

Dose. Lithium carbonate should be begun at 600–900 mg per day in divided doses of 300 mg each. The sustained-release preparations (e.g., Eskalith CR, Lithobid) should not be used at this stage of treatment, although they may be more convenient for maintenance. A liquid form, lithium citrate, is also available.

Serum lithium levels should be checked twice a week after beginning treatment, and the dose increased every few days until about 0.7–1.2 mEq per liter is attained. Lithium levels should be obtained in the morning, before the first dose (and at least 10 hours after the last dose).

Although there is some variability in patient response, serum lithium levels below 0.7 mEq/1 are unlikely to be helpful in acute stages. Levels above 1.2 mEq/1 and up to 1.5 mEq/1 may be needed in treatment of acute mania; however, many patients develop toxic signs at this dose. Levels should not be allowed to exceed 1.5 mEq/1. Most patients will reach therapeutic serum levels at 900–1800 mg of lithium carbonate ($LiCO_3$) per day.

One may slowly increase the lithium over one or two weeks to the dose that results in therapeutic levels, but several other ways of predicting the eventual lithium dose have been reported. These generally suggest a loading dose followed by serial lithium levels over 24 hours. Zetin et al. (1986) have developed a "mathematical alternative" to the loading-dose method. At this time, the trial-and-error method seems easy and quite satisfactory in most settings.

Combining lithium with neuroleptic medication is considered safe and clinically appropriate for many manic patients who do not respond to lithium alone. The patient should be monitored closely, however, and significant increases in the dose of either drug should be followed by monitoring of the lithium level (e.g., at three days and 10 days post-increase). If a severe adverse reaction should occur, both drugs should be stopped, medical support promptly initiated, electrolytes closely monitored, and the patient treated as one would treat neuroleptic malignant syndrome (q.v.) until clinical condition dictates otherwise.

Lithium side effects. Mild tremor, mild gastric upset, and increased thirst (accompanied by appropriately increased urinary output) are the most common side effects. They may be seen in patients whose lithium levels are well below the toxic range. The dose may be adjusted to decrease side effects while retaining therapeutic effect. Extrapyramidal symptoms occasionally occur. A few patients complain of memory problems. Weight gain is not unusual, whether from increased appetite (perhaps because of the patient's improved psychiatric condition) or lithium-induced edema. Temporary hypothyroidism is routine and should not be treated unless clinical symptoms occur. Thyroid supplements can usually be discontinued after a few weeks, if they are needed in the first place.

In spite of traditional concerns about combining lithium with thiazide diuretics, cautious addition of a thiazide diuretic to control benign polyuria can allow some patients who truly need lithium treatment to continue it safely. When this is done, *the lithium dose should be decreased by 50%, and the lithium level restabilized.* The clinician must remember that lithium is a salt whose concentration and bioavailability is closely linked to that of sodium (and to some extent potassium) (see Patient Instructions, p. 208).

Other side effects, mostly rare, include benign skin rashes (which may disappear if the brand is changed), exacerbation of psoriasis, altered glucose tolerance test (Shah et al., 1986), Graves' disease (or the masking of Graves' disease) (Thompson & Baylis, 1986), self-limited alopecia (Ghadirian & Lalinec-Michaud, 1986), and a variety of benign renal effects (see below) (Vaamonde et al., 1986).

Serious adverse effects of lithium are almost always related to toxicity. Although the toxic level for this drug is quite close to the therapeutic level, serum levels tend to be stable, with the following exceptions:

1. Acute electrolyte imbalance, usually caused by significant vomiting, diarrhea, or other fluid loss, rapidly increasing the serum lithium level.
2. Ingestion of medications, almost always physician-prescribed, which alter electrolyte balance. Diuretics are the most obvious offenders; however, ibuprofen (Ragheb, 1987) and other drugs increase lithium levels to a variable extent in many patients.
3. Anything that decreases glomerular filtration rates and lithium clearance through the kidney, increasing serum lithium levels. Some examples are found in elderly patients (Greil et al., 1985; Vestergaard & Schou, 1984) and pregnant patients (Kaufman & Okeya, 1985)
4. Dietary salt restriction. Patients should be cautioned to include normal amounts of salt in their daily diets. Although no added

salt is necessary, patients beginning low-or no-salt diets (or unusual or "fad" diets) should have their lithium levels re-stabilized.

Early reports of *renal* damage from chronic lithium prescription have been replaced by many studies that indicate little or no danger of irreversible renal impairment (e.g., glomerular damage) (DePaulo, Correau, & Sapir, 1986; Vaamonde et al., 1986). Because of effects on *thyroid* function, a few studies have been done that indicate possible fluctuations in thyroid immune status on chronic lithium carbonate therapy (Lazarus et al., 1986). There is a small but measurable rate of development of persistent *tardive dyskinesia* in bipolar patients. Most such cases involve patients who have taken neuroleptics at some point (Mukherjee et al., 1986; Perenyi, Szuchs, & Frecska, 1984). This danger is not felt to be significant enough to warrant specific warnings to patients receiving lithium alone.

Lithium therapy should be continued only with caution in *pregnant patients*, particularly in the first trimester. The risk:benefit ratio may be acceptable for many patients, since symptomatic bipolar illness can be dangerous to both the woman and the fetus. The many physiological changes of pregnancy make close monitoring and restabilization of the lithium level necessary. Lithium should be discontinued well before delivery (Jefferson, Greist, & Ackerman, 1983). Breast-feeding should be discouraged, since lithium easily passes into breast milk.

Treatment of lithium toxicity and overdose. Ordinary toxicity is treated very simply, by withholding one or more doses of the drug. In the absence of renal complications, it is rapidly cleared. Serious toxicity, such as that associated with overdose (which may produce acute renal failure) can be treated with hemodialysis, over several days if necessary (Fenves, Emmettt, & White, 1984; Jaeger et al., 1985).

Patient instructions. Patients should be carefully told, orally and in writing, about the special characteristics of lithium carbonate, especially compared to other commonly prescribed psychotropic drugs. Patients are often accustomed to medications whose blood levels are not closely monitored, and whose therapeutic-to-toxic-level ratio is fairly low. There are a number of patient information sheets commercially available, including one from the American Medical Association.

The patient should be cautioned not to alter the dose, to maintain a normal dietary salt intake, to report for scheduled lithium level monitoring, to communicate to other physicians that he or she is taking lithium (and tell the psychiatrist if other drugs are prescribed), and to call the psychiatrist if serious vomiting, diarrhea, or other fluid loss occurs. The patient should be instructed to skip a lithium dose if toxic signs arise or fluid or electrolyte loss occurs, especially if he or she is unable to contact the doctor or clinic.

Patients with Manic or Mixed Bipolar Disorder are often concerned about how their treatment will affect the feelings of well-being, creativity, or social and professional success that have often been present for many years before their first "break." It is useful to tell them that, unlike some of the medications used for serious psychiatric illness, lithium is not an emotional "downer," nor is it known to affect normal energy or creativity. The lay impression of lithium as a "mood stabilizer" is a useful one, implying that the patient remains free to experience the normal emotions of life, but is protected from destructive or bizarre swings of mood.

Acute hospital settings. Although the patient may not appear amenable to logic or verbal approaches, a structured setting is important. The staff should be familiar with treatment methods for agitated or highly active patients, as well as with signs of lithium toxicity.

As the acute symptoms subside, discharge plans should be formulated which stress the biological, psychological, and social needs of the patient. Education of the patient and significant others about the special characteristics of bipolar illness (in addition to the characteristics of lithium carbonate, mentioned above) is important, since relapse of hypomania or mania is not usually associated with dysphoric warning signs.

Maintenance Treatment. Careful discharge planning and attention to the transition from inpatient to outpatient care are the keys to lasting psychiatric and social post-hospital success. Care should be taken to help the patient with his or her first contact with the outpatient environment: for example, providing for visits from the therapist (or visits to the outpatient clinic) while the patient is still in the hospital. At the least, the name and location of the follow-up therapist, a scheduled appointment, and a written description of medications and dosages should be in the patient's hands before he or she leaves the hospital.

Most bipolar patients do not require chronic medication other than lithium to remain in remission. Neuroleptics can usually be discontinued before the patient leaves the hospital, or soon thereafter. It is poor practice to discontinue the neuroleptic just as the patient is discharged (or, for that matter, to make any major changes in the medication regimen during this transition period). Even if it is pharmacologically unnecessary, one should wait until the outpatient situation is stabilized before proceeding to discontinue the neuroleptic.

The lithium itself is crucial to preventing relapse. It should not be discontinued without careful supervision. Most patients require treatment for an indefinite period.

Patients on maintenance lithium may be able to remain in remission at serum levels below those required for acute treatment. Most clinicians prefer serum levels above about 0.6 mEq/l (Maj et al., 1986). There are patients who can remain in remission at levels as low as 0.4 mEq/l; however, it seems imprudent to allow this in the absence of unusual dose-related side effects.

Prognosis and Outcome. The prognosis for lithium-responding manic or mixed bipolar patients is generally good, provided they remain in treatment and lithium levels can be reasonably monitored (at least every three months once the patient is completely stable). A large collaborative study (Prien et al., 1984) showed no advantage of drug combinations over lithium carbonate alone in maintenance treatment.

Relapse rate is correlated with a number of clinical factors. Goodnick and colleagues (1987) found response to lithium prophylaxis largely determined by frequency of manic or depressive episodes and duration of lithium treatment. Others find few predictors of outcome based upon clinical factors alone (Mander, 1986). Keller and colleagues (1986) found that bipolar manic patients were considerably more likely to remain free of illness after treatment than either mixed or purely depressed patients. Finally, a Danish population study followed bipolar and un-ipolar "manic depressive" patients and compared them with the general population, finding that all patients with the "manic depressive" illness had increased mortality by suicide and accidents, and that the bipolar group had a higher mortality from nonviolent causes than the unipolar group (Weeke & Vaeth, 1986).

Alternative Biological Therapies. Refractory manic psychosis or rapid cycling of manic–depressive psychosis can often be successfully treated with ECT (Berman & Wolpert, 1987). (Guidelines are summarized on pp. 234–237)

Folic acid supplements, up to 200 mcg per day, may add to the ability of lithium to prevent return of affective illness. In one study, patients for whom this supplement actually increased plasma folate to 13 ng/ml or above had significant reduction in affective morbidity. Some authors suggest a daily supplement of 300–400 mcg (Coppen, Chaudhry, & Swade, 1986).

The use of *depot neuroleptics* in patients with poor lithium prophylaxis or psychotic symptoms between manic episodes has been recommended by several authors (Lowe & Batchelor, 1986). Both fluphenazine decanoate and haloperidol decanoate have been used. The doses are usually about the same as, or lower than, doses required for control of schizophrenia. Maintenance should be at the lowest effective dose, since affective illness has been associated with increased risk of tardive dyskinesia in patients taking neuroleptics.

Adding *carbamazepine* to the lithium regimen has often been found superior to lithium alone or combinations of lithium and neuroleptics, particularly in maintenance treatment (Shukla, Cook, & Miller, 1985). Carbamazepine alone also has an antimanic effect and some ability to prevent recurrent depression (Lerer et al., 1987; Stromgren & Boller, 1985). The clinician should be familiar with the prescription information and cautions regarding blood count before proceeding.

The calcium channel blocker *verapamil* has also been studied and found to have some antimanic activity. When available, it may be useful for patients unable to take lithium (Dubovsky et al., 1986; Solomon & Williamson, 1986). When verapamil is given with lithium, there is apparently increased danger of neurotoxicity (Price & Giannini, 1986). *Sodium valproate* has both an acute antimanic effect and prophylactic action, as does *oxcarbazepine*, a relative of carbamazepine (Emrich, Dose, & von Zerssen, 1985). Of all these alternatives to lithium, carbamazepine is felt to be the most reliable (Lerer, 1985).

Finally, acute treatment of manic agitation with *lorazepam* (Lenox, Modell, & Weiner, 1986) and other benzodiazepines may have not only a sedative, but also an antipsychotic effect. These medications are generally quite safe, rarely mask other symptoms, and act rapidly; however, they should not be considered for definitive treatment or prophylaxis of mania.

Psychosocial Treatments in Manic and Mixed Bipolar Disorder. Even in highly medical settings, combined psychopharmacologic and psychodynamic therapies are more useful in the long run than biological therapies alone. The "biopsychosocial" approach is too often overlooked by psychiatrists, particularly in academic or busy clinical settings. Personality characteristics of recovered patients, for example, differ sub-

Related Psychosocial Disorders. The treatment of psychiatric or psychosocial problems that may accompany post-traumatic syndromes is an important part of total care. Two of the most common are depression and substance abuse.

Depression frequently remits with psychotherapy of PTSD, but should be vigorously treated if it remains behind when other symptoms remit. Substance abuse disorders are considerably more complex, and should usually be treated as if they were primary. That is, the clinician should not expect the substance abuse to disappear with psychotherapy for the Post-traumatic Stress Disorder (and, conversely, the substance abuse treatment program should specifically address PTSD). Increasing self-image, decreasing guilt, and reexperiencing and reintegrating the trauma are common parts of combined substance abuse/PTSD treatment programs for, for example, Vietnam veterans (Jelinek & Williams, 1984; Schnitt & Nocks, 1984).

Finally, many PTSD patients, particularly combat veterans or victims of mass disasters, benefit from lay support groups. Where possible, these groups should have the benefit of psychiatric consultation or participation.

300.02 Generalized Anxiety Disorder

A recent controlled trial of treatments for generalized anxiety (Lindsay et al., 1987) found that although anxiolytic drugs (benzodiazepines) were rapidly and significantly effective at reducing anxiety early in treatment, groups receiving drugs alone tended quickly to relapse. The most significant and consistent improvements were seen in groups receiving cognitive-behavioral therapy or anxiety management training. Nevertheless, most patients who reach the physician's (including the psychiatrist's) office receive anxiolytic medication, and perhaps brief psychotherapy. Choice of drug and dosage schedule should be clearly separated from medication for panic attacks or relief of acute anxiety.

Drug Treatment. Benzodiazepines are the anxiolytics of choice. Treatment may take two forms. First, the medication may be prescribed with the understanding that it will be available for only a short time, while psychotherapy, behavioral treatment, or merely the passage of time remove the source of generalized anxiety. Because of development of tolerance, medication abuse, potential physical dependence, and the long half-life of several of these drugs (e.g., diazepam), the short-half-life benzodiazepines (e.g., oxazepam) are preferred. In spite of many cautions, particularly in the lay literature, benzodiazepines are very effective, quite safe in both therapeutic regimen and overdose, have excellent patient acceptance, and cause few side effects. Except for side-effects profile and half-life, all of the common benzodiazepines, including alprazolam, are similarly effective (Cordingley, Dean, & Hallett, 1985; Dunner et al., 1986; Fontaine et al., 1986).

Reid (1983) suggests a second approach, in which the benzodiazepine need not actually be ingested in order for it to contribute to the patient's improvement. Formation of a therapeutic relationship with a patient often allows therapeutic reassurance and the mere carrying of the medication (perhaps as symbolic representations of the therapist) to supplant the chronic taking of drugs. In this plan, the medication is prescribed on a per-day or per-week basis (e.g., two tablets per day, or 10 tablets per week, no matter when they are taken) rather than in a fixed schedule. This is a logical way to prescribe for Panic Disorder (see p. 246), if one is using benzodiazepines, as well.

Some of the benzodiazepines, notably clorazepate (Zung, 1987) and alprazolam, are said to be effective for depressed mood in patients who are anxious. Careful evaluation of the patient should allow one to separate primary affective disorder with anxiety from primary anxiety disorder with concomitant depression.

Buspirone. The first nonbenzodiazepine anxiolytic to be introduced for many years, buspirone has been heavily studied, but has had insufficient clinical exposure to conclusively establish its usefulness in the U.S. The primary indication for buspirone is chronic or generalized anxiety without panic attacks. It acts quite slowly, often taking two to three weeks for complete effect.

One should begin with small doses, around 5 mg twice a day, increasing to 20–30 mg per day within the first week to 10 days. It has little or no immediate effect, and thus should not be used for acute relief or as-needed anxiolytic treatment. Patients notice little or no medication effect, and should not expect to feel better immediately. Interestingly, patients who have been taking benzodiazepines usually respond poorly to buspirone. Whether this is a pharmacologic effect or is related to buspirone's not providing any immediate feeling of well-being is not clear.

Buspirone provides some advantages, and a couple of disadvantages, in comparison to other anxiolytics (including meprobamate or barbiturates). It apparently has little or no interaction with or potentiation of alcohol or other CNS depressants. It is thus far not known to have a potential for tolerance or physical dependence, and is unlikely to encourage emotional dependence. It is apparently fairly safe in overdose. It does not block the withdrawal effects of alcohol, benzodiazepines, meprobamate, or sedatives/hypnotics, and has little or no anticonvulsant activity. Side effects are occasional and generally benign, including dizziness, headache, nervousness, and lightheadedness (*International Drug Therapy Newsletter*, 1984; Newton et al., 1986).

Other Nonbenzodiazepines. Hydroxyzine is a useful anxiolytic but is somewhat sedative and anticholinergic. Meprobamate, once commonly prescribed for anxiety, is a poor choice because of its limited effectiveness, high addictive potential, and serious withdrawal syndrome.

Some experimental medications, as well as some drugs currently experimental for generalized anxiety, should be briefly mentioned. The tricyclic and MAOI antidepressants have both been prescribed, although they are probably more indicated for primary blockade of panic disorder than for chronic anxiety. Atenolol has been studied outside the U.S. (Saul et al., 1985), as have the benzodiazepine methylclonazepam (Ansseau et al., 1985) and a buspirone relative, gepirone (Csanalosi et al., 1987), all with some success.

Psychotherapy. It is often effective for the therapist to inform the patient that although this condition is quite uncomfortable, it has predictable patterns (and is thus potentially understandable) and is quite separate from more serious, "psychotic" mental illness. The possibility of frequent relapse should be frankly addressed as part of reassurance that the course of the disorder is fairly predictable and is likely to improve with time. As with Panic Disorder (p. 246) intensive or psychoanalytic psychotherapy may be helpful for a few patients; however, it is usually not cost-effective unless there are clear underlying conflicts which the patient is motivated to address, and for which the patient can tolerate psychodynamic exploration.

Many patients with Generalized Anxiety Disorder have personality characteristics or coping styles that must be considered as one shapes the psychotherapeutic plan. Some have anxiety accompanied by considerable dependency or clinging to the clinician. Specific rules for when and how the therapist will be available may alleviate some of the therapist's discomfort and provide an atmosphere of consistency for the patient. It is unreasonable, and usually countertherapeutic, to be so "available" to the patient that he or she is encouraged to call whenever symptoms arise.

Cognitive and Behavioral Treatments. Relaxation training, desensitization, biofeedback, and "stress inoculation" have all been used successfully, with and without medication, for the short-term treatment of anxiety disorders. Relaxation therapy (often including training the patient to carry out the therapy himself or herself) and other, behavioral methods for giving the patient control over his or her anxiety tend to be associated with continued improvement months or years later (Holcomb, 1986; Spencer, 1986; Tarrier & Main, 1986).

Other Treatments. Inhalation of carbon dioxide (diluted with air but in concentrations well above normal expiration) has long been known to alleviate anxiety and "hyperventilation." There is now at least behavioral evidence that carbon dioxide inhalation may provide anxiety reduction which lasts up to several weeks, perhaps because of an operant conditioning effect: weakening of the anxiety response by competitive response to carbon dioxide (Wolpe, 1987). Anecdotal evidence for its effectiveness is frequently reported, with occasional controlled studies (Lanza, 1986). An ancient Chinese remedy, suanzaorentang, was recently studied in a double-blind clinical trial and found to possess anxiolytic effects comparable to diazepam, in doses of 750 mg per day (Chen, Hsie, & Shibuya, 1986).

300.00 Anxiety Disorder Not Otherwise Specified

The treatment of other anxiety disorders should be predicated upon the symptoms presented and the underlying situational and psychodynamic issues elicited during evaluation. Many of the principles mentioned in this chapter may apply. Practical counseling, in an atmosphere of support and reassurance, is a good adjunct to any treatment program. An understanding of the patient's personality or character style, as well as careful evaluation for medical or environmental correlates, increases the opportunity for treatment success.

Chapter 19

Somatoform Disorders

300.70 Body Dysmorphic Disorder (Dysmorphophobia)
300.70 Hypochondriasis (Hypochondriacal Neurosis)
In this section we will discuss the two above disorders together, since there are many similarities and insufficient differentiation in the modern treatment literature to separate them. Similarities in treatment concept with the several other somatoform disorders are apparent as well; the reader is encouraged to examine this entire Somatoform Disorders section for suggestions related to treatment of individual patients with any of these diagnoses.

Two issues that must be addressed before treating a patient for primary hypochondria are the adequate exclusion of medical illness (including brain disease which manifests as delusions of bodily symptoms or dysmorphia) (Takeda et al., 1985) and treatment of accompanying psychiatric disorders which may be giving rise to the anxieties, obsessions, or delusions of bodily disease. The symptomatic treatments below are unlikely to be helpful for patients in whom the source of the illness behavior is, for example, a guilt-ridden depression or a paranoid psychosis.

A practical means for the primary physician to treat hypochondriasis and several other somatoform disorders is described by Kellner (1982a). Patients are given accurate information about the interaction between their emotions and possible physical symptoms; the benign nature of the somatoform disorder is emphasized; and the fact that there is a good medical prognosis is celebrated by the physician. Good physical examinations are performed and the patient is allowed to have regular, brief physician visits. The patient is not allowed to expand his illness behavior into frequent, "as-needed" medical calls, but is strongly encouraged and reassured that he has a consistent place in the physician's appointment schedule.

In hypochondriasis, and to some extent in the other somatoform disorders, concern over loss of the physician (and the object that the physician symbolizes) can be a significant impediment to lasting improvement. Thus, the physician who tells the patient "I have good news. Your tests are all negative. You don't need to come back and see me" may well precipitate further symptoms or complaints which are designed to recover the lost physician or object.

Individual psychotherapy that focuses on the here-and-now complaints, fears, and beliefs of the patient is frequently successful, with good long-term outcome associated with fairly brief symptom duration and the absence of a personality disorder diagnosis. Outcome is not particularly associated with age, sex, severity of symptoms, or severity of anxiety (Kellner, 1983). Psychotropic drugs are effective in reducing anxiety, and for treating patients with mixed psychiatric disorders (Kellner, 1985).

Although patients with somatoform disorders are often felt to be difficult to treat with psychotherapy, when both the primary physician and the psychotherapist can communicate their understanding of the patient's distress, he or she can be engaged in treatment (Galatzer-Levy, 1982). The presence of the psychiatrist as part of a medical team emphasizes the integration of psychiatric issues with medical fears and symptoms.

Traditional insight-oriented psychotherapy can be helpful for patients whose hypochondriasis is symptomatic of neurotic conflict, and who are willing to engage in it. Once the patient has entered treatment, it may be useful to discourage talk about the hypochondriacal symptoms during certain phases of therapy, with the idea that this topic is a resistance and prevents the surfacing of other important material.

Group therapy is a cost-effective alternative to individual psychotherapy or visits to the primary physician, and can provide ventilation, interpersonal relationships, and help with dependency needs.

The source of the illness behavior can be a form of manipulating others or responding to stress, for example, in a patient who wishes to generate guilt in others or bring them closer to him or her. These reasons can be used to develop a psychosocial treatment program which may include the patient, the family, and training in other ways to accomplish the needed aggression, attention, or caring from others. A few behavioral protocols have been described for treating hypochondriasis, disordered body image, or disease phobia. The most common is exposure, which treats the disorder as a phobia (Tearnan et al., 1985).

Monosymptomatic Hypochondriasis. The obsession with a particular serious physical disorder or symptom, such as a delusionally aberrant body image, body smell, internal parasite, or malformation, is frequently associated with a severe personality disorder, psychosis, or organic central nervous system deficit. Evaluation should be vigorous, particularly if one of the senses (e.g., smell, taste, touch) is involved. Treatment often requires antipsychotic medication, even if a brain lesion is present. The high-potency drugs, such as haloperidol (Andrews, Bellard, & Walter-Ryan, 1986) or (outside the U.S.) pimozide, may be helpful.

When talking of disorders of body image or obsessions with bodily defects, it is important that a differentiation be made between patients with a somatoform disorder and those with eating disorders (Anorexia Nervosa, Bulimia Nervosa) or Transsexualism, all of which are addressed elsewhere in this text.

300.11 Conversion Disorder (Hysterical Neurosis, Conversion Type)

Conversion reactions often disappear of their own accord in hours or days—sometimes in response to lost opportunities for secondary gain. In some cases the rapid loss of symptoms is misunderstood as always connoting "malingering."

Response to symptomatic treatment is usually quite good. If symptom removal is the only goal of treatment, then hypnosis or behavior therapy should be considered. Simple suggestion or "magical" symptom removal through amytal interview or other clinical trickery should usually be avoided, and treatment provided in a broader context. Particular attention should be given to making improvement permanent, generalizing it to other maladaptive ways of handling the underlying conflicts that gave rise to the physical symptom.

Suggestion or amytal interview may be used for diagnostic purposes, although mere disappearance of symptoms is not conclusive evidence of their functional origin. The psychiatrist may thus assist when conversion patients present in a general hospital setting, by helping to differentiate conversion from organic symptoms or malingering, and by educating the hospital staff in methods of humane management and approaches to the patient (e.g., discouraging direct confrontation or accusations by staff) (Cohen et al., 1985; Lazara, 1981).

The clinician should establish himself as someone who has genuine respect for the patient and his or her difficulties. He should have a medical background, since up to 25% of patients originally diagnosed by nonpsychiatric physicians to have conversion disorders are eventually found to have organic disease, often of a degenerative type (Watson & Buranen, 1979).

Involvement of the spouse and/or other important family members in the patient's care, with an understanding of the social and psychodynamic issues that may be involved, can promote better communication and decrease the need for future conversion symptoms.

If the patient has a true hysterical neurosis, intensive or psychoanalytic psychotherapy is indicated. Unfortunately, conversion symptoms are nonspecific, and patients with more severe underlying pathology (e.g., personality disorders) may appear clinically similar to those with hysterical neurosis before treatment is begun (Shalev & Munitz, 1986). For those patients, dynamic psychotherapy may help with symptoms but is usually not the best approach in the long run.

Patients with good premorbid adjustment, absence of major psychiatric syndromes, and the presence of a stressful event associated with acute onset of the conversion symptoms are associated with good prognosis. Most patients without severe underlying psychopathology continue to be significantly improved several years after treatment, although for some the conversion reaction is an indicator of ongoing emotional problems or, as mentioned above, developing physical disease.

300.81 Somatization Disorder
(See also Somatoform Pain Disorder—307.80.)
The first tenet of treatment is understanding that patients with Somatization Disorder (or Briquet's syndrome) are not immune from physical illness. It is a serious mistake for any physician, much less a psychiatrist, to underestimate the patient's symptoms and the discomfort that they are causing, or to label them using discriminatory terms (e.g., "crock"). Excellent diagnostic procedures are usually possible without invasive techniques. Excessive medical care is expensive, however, sometimes dangerous, and can usually be avoided (Ries et al., 1981; Zoccolillo & Cloninger, 1986).

There are a number of clinical approaches to the somatizing patient (including those represented among the other somatoform disorders). The primary physician can manage many, if not most, of these patients by developing a good physician–patient relationship, applying rudimentary techniques of behavior modification, expanding the patient's care to include attention to life stresses, treating symptoms conservatively, watching for depression, and understanding the importance of ongoing contact with the patient (Smith, 1985).

The psychiatrist in a consultation-liaison setting can help the non-psychiatric treatment team both understand the patient's complaints and, perhaps more importantly, understand the concept that because these patients cling to their symptoms for emotional reasons, "care" rather than "cure" is the cornerstone of management (Lichstein, 1986).

Symptomatic outpatient follow-up is recommended for those patients who are willing to engage in psychotherapy. A number of techniques are helpful, including short-term, anxiety-provoking psychotherapy (Sifneos, 1984), relaxation therapy (Johnson, Shenoy, & Langer, 1981), combination approaches such as the coping-rest model (Moss & Garb, 1986), and reality- and insight-oriented group psychotherapies (Schreter, 1980). Each should provide support and mild, tolerable confrontation. In both group and individual therapy, the clinician should be alert for nonsomatic symptoms of underlying conflict (e.g., depression), and be prepared to recognize and treat them accordingly.

Definitive treatment of Somatization Disorder involves the removal of the emotional precursors of multiple medical complaints and/or the channeling of coping mechanisms for those precursors into behaviors or emotions that are more effective for the patient than are the symptoms of Somatization Disorder. Unfortunately, most clinicians report only limited success for traditional psychodynamic intervention (Karasu, 1979; Kellner, 1975).

Karasu (1979) recommends that the psychotherapist relate to the patient as a physician to a medically ill individual, well informed about the patient's illness. Once this empathy and understanding have been established, a "life alliance" promotes friendly and educational interactions. After several weeks, the patient may eventually be able to explore feelings toward the therapist, feelings toward the symptoms, and the possibility that these are related. Once the patient has meaningful insight into the relationships among affect, behavior, and somatization, symptoms of anxiety or physical distress should lessen. Nevertheless, patients who have expressed feelings in terms of bodily sensation may, by definition, be those who are reluctant to accept a psychotherapeutic approach.

In the absence of serious underlying psychiatric illness, the use of medications to treat this and similar somatoform disorders is not recommended. On the other hand, the psychiatrist should remain aware that somatic symptoms can be atypical presentations of, for example, depression.

307.80   Somatoform Pain Disorder

This disorder, called Psychogenic Pain Disorder in *DSM-III*, should be viewed multidimensionally (Getto & Ochitill, 1982). This places the psychiatrist treating a somatoform disorder into the multidisciplinary group of physicians and others who have a common goal of alleviating and preventing the patient's pain. One important aspect of this approach is that it may allow the patient to accept psychiatric intervention more readily in a situation that the patient perceives as nonpsychiatric.

Another important part of treatment is the clinician's belief that the patient actually feels pain and requires treatment. This—and the corollary belief that the patient is being honest with the physician— may be lacking in many of the patient's previous interactions with physicians. This does not preclude the psychiatrist's expressing his or her belief that even very considerable pain can begin in, and be mediated by, the human mind.

The psychiatrist should be a person who works well within medical settings and is comfortable discussing and evaluating medical illness in his or her patients (Murphy & Davis, 1981). The dual orientations of medicine and psychology offer reassurance that the patient continues to be medically monitored.

One view of Somatoform Pain Disorder compares it to other forms of chronic pain, and recommends treatment along similar lines. Pain clinics, usually found in larger medical institutions, use clear guidelines for evaluation, treatment goals, and attaining those goals. This struc- turing activity, often in an inpatient setting, transforms a confusing and overwhelming pain experience into one with manageable parts. The patient participates in the program to a great extent, and thereby gains some measure of mastery over feelings and sensations toward which he or she was formerly passive.

The programs are primarily behavioral, with reinforcement for decreasing "pain behavior" as well as for the more obvious goals of decreased use of medication and lessened perception of pain. Biofeed- back and group therapy are often used. Since the chronic pain takes place in, and is part of, the patient's family and social life, attention must be paid to education and counseling for the family and preparation for activities of daily living. Such programs generally last for several weeks or months, and frequently have high success rates among patients who have not done well with previous (usually drug-oriented) regimens.

Treatment is sometimes criticized for its emphasis on simply decreasing hospital visits and demands on the physician's time. Such goals should, however, be seen as being attained because the pain behavior is no longer necessary from the patient's viewpoint, and not merely as the result of "punishment" for visiting the clinic. Indeed, reassurance that the doctor and other means of alleviating pain are available is a large part of showing the patient that he or she does not need to *use* the medical facilities to prove that they are there.

Many forms of chronic pain are treated with tricyclic antidepressants and some other psychotropic medications. In some reports, psychogenic pain responds as well. The best patient response often occurs at doses consistent with antidepressant activity; however, it has not been shown that effectiveness of the medication is due to its antidepressant qualities. Some recommend the tricyclics as an early choice, before resorting to inpatient pain control programs.

It is virtually impossible to change severe, often personality-related pain behavior, usually associated with secondary gain, in an outpatient setting. Insight-oriented psychodynamic psychotherapy is not often a treatment of choice, and when applied should carefully isolate the pain symptom from the bulk of the verbal therapy. Supportive therapy may seem helpful, and may serve to keep the patient functioning in his or her social environment, but generally has little more than superficial value.

300.70 Undifferentiated Somatoform Disorder
300.70 Somatoform Disorder Not Otherwise Specified

The treatment of Undifferentiated Somatoform Disorder or Somatoform Disorder Not Otherwise Specified should be based upon the principles already outlined in this section, the presenting symptoms, and the clinician's understanding of the underlying medical and psychological disorders.

Chapter 20

Dissociative Disorders (Hysterical Neuroses, Dissociative Type)

300.14 Multiple Personality Disorder

The treatment of this rare disorder is far more complex and lengthy than that of any of the other, relatively encapsulated dissociative disorders. The condition should not be considered synonymous with schizophreniform disorders, and should not be treated with antipsychotic medication unless indicated by the symptoms presented. The traditional approach, popularized by Thigpen and Cleckley (1957), is intensely psychodynamic or psychoanalytic, often aided by hypnosis. The hypnotic portion of treatment may be used to uncover material for therapeutic exploration outside the trance or, if the clinician is trained in the psychoanalytic use of trance, may be an aid to restructuring the patient's character in such a way as to integrate the various separated parts, each of which is incomplete without the others.

The psychotherapeutic treatment of multiple personality requires sufficient subspecialization that the clinician should either be experienced in this area or seek supervision. The patient, with his or her various, often uncooperative parts, will tend to be demanding and frustrating. Nevertheless, many clinicians feel that when understood as a chronic dissociative Post-traumatic Stress Disorder—that is, arising out of intolerable childhood traumata—Multiple Personality Disorder has an excellent prognosis if treated by an experienced clinician using intensive, prolonged psychotherapy (Kluft, 1987).

The recent marked increase in reported cases of multiple personality patients is difficult to explain. This author believes that much of the increase is related to the "popularity" of the disorder, and particularly its popularity among certain therapists who "specialize" in its treatment. Considerable caution with respect to diagnosis and treatment is indicated for at least the following reasons.

1. Focus on the "multiple personality" aspects of the patient as his or her most interesting characteristics and as sources of extra attention from the therapist creates a setting in which the often highly suggestible patient unconsciously creates (or worsens, by adding additional parts) the very disease being treated. This is especially likely with hypnotic treatments in relatively inexperienced hands (see below).
2. The therapist may be seduced by the notoriety—among other professionals, patients, or the public—of treating these exotic individuals.
3. Individual, especially legal, responsibility for one's actions may be questioned or avoided altogether. Whether or not the patient has Multiple Personality Disorder, to exonerate him from responsibility for his actions is often inappropriate and almost always countertherapeutic.
4. Serious countertransference reactions, including anger, exasperation, exhaustion, and even sexual seduction or violence are not uncommon (Coons, 1986a; Watkins & Watkins, 1984).

Because Multiple Personality Disorder is commonly felt to represent a chronic, global reaction to childhood trauma, some authors suggest early, even childhood diagnosis and treatment (Coons, 1986b).

Hypnotic Treatments. It has long been recognized that patients with dissociative disorders are easily hypnotizable. Spiegel (1984) notes multiple personality patients' spontaneous dissociation to protect themselves from emotional and physical pain. Bliss (1980) even suggests that the core of multiple personality is in unrecognized self-hypnosis, by which the patient has created a number of personalities and allowed experiences or functions to be delegated to alter egos.

Using hypnosis as a means for communicating with and eventually integrating the parts of the patient's personality (which should be clearly understood as *parts*, and not separate personalities) raises the danger that either the therapist or the patient will actually create new parts or "personalities" in response to the highly suggestible emotional milieu. The danger is exacerbated by trance and by the strong implication that the therapist expects, and will be gratified by, the uncovering of additional "personalities."

The process of uncovering, appearing to uncover, or communicating with parts of the personality in trance and then suggesting that they will be remembered by, and integrated with, the dominant personality is simplistic and incomplete. The patient must see his or her parts as parts of an already existing "whole." It is probably countertherapeutic even to refer to each part by a separate name. If this seems unavoidable, one should make it clear that the names are merely labels, and do not connote any acceptance by the therapist that the patient actually contains more than one "person."

No matter what the psychotherapeutic treatment choice, resistances related to repression, denial, secrecy, and crises that threaten to disintegrate the treatment process must be addressed (Coons, 1986a). The anxiety-ridden perceptions, memories, and screened memories that have given rise to dissociative and depressive symptoms must be dealt with, and more adaptive resolutions found. In particular, depression and loss may need to be addressed with either psychotherapy or biological approaches as treatment progresses.

Restraint. A word should be added about the therapeutic use of physical restraint suggested by a few authors (Young, 1986). This technique suggests voluntary, intermittent use of restraints to work through "dangerous" situations of the bringing out and treatment of angry or aggressive parts of the personality, with the aim of providing a physically and emotionally safe environment for both patient and therapist.

This author would suggest great caution in this and other abreactive techniques, and recommends experienced supervision if it is attempted. There is considerable danger of (1) creating a "special" setting for this "special" and potentially gratifying symptom, (2) creating considerable potential for patient abuse and sensationalism, and (3) creating a seductive, "secret" affect-laden experience with the therapist.

300.13   Psychogenic Fugue

Psychogenic Fugue may be considered similar in purpose to amnesia but as involving a necessity for more dissociation from an affect-laden event and/or from the self. Many of the treatment techniques described in the next section on Psychogenic Amnesia are useful for fugue. The clinician should expect treatment to be more lengthy, consistent with the more massive defensive mechanism (or with a premorbid character structure which was predisposed to it). Since Psychogenic Fugue may last longer than amnesia, therapeutic strategies that include more intense psychodynamic therapy are often suggested. At the least, a continuing supportive relationship with a psychotherapist is recommended for preventing future dissociative episodes.

Many treatment techniques, particularly hypnosis and amytal interview, are aimed at recovering the patient's memory for things that happened during the fugue state. As was implied in the previous section on multiple personality, caution should be used when hypnotic techniques are used to "reconstruct" memory, since what may appear to be restitution of old memory is often actually construction of new "memory" (Orne, 1979). In some patients, this is not a significant problem; however, when the recovering of a specific memory is important (e.g., for legal reasons), hypnosis should be used only with the greatest of care in order to assure that the "memory" is not actually an iatrogenic confabulation which becomes permanently imbedded in the patient's past.

Symptom-oriented approaches such as hypnosis, amytal interview, or even brief psychotherapy sometimes imply that the patient's symptoms are interesting and worth keeping because of the attention they generate. When possible, psychotherapeutic approaches should try to uncover the stressful and conflictual sources of the fugue, and provide alternative needs for dealing with the painful affects against which fugue is a defense.

300.12   Psychogenic Amnesia

The most common clinical presentation of Psychogenic Amnesia is in an emergency room or military clinic, often following severe emotional trauma (which may be accompanied by physical injury). In spite of the fact that Psychogenic Amnesia frequently clears without treatment, early intervention to prevent stabilization of the amnesia and its incorporation into the patient's emotional structure is recommended.

Both active and passive treatment methods have been advocated. Since amnesia produces anxiety in family and friends, there is usually pressure to alleviate it quickly. Barbiturate interviews and hypnotic techniques often give access to the suppressed memories.

One may suggest that the patient will recall the events upon arousal; however, most clinicians prefer to allow the *patient* to make this decision, saying something like: "When you become alert, you will be able to remember as much of our interview as you like; the rest will come to you in time, when you are ready to recall it." This allows the mind to use the amnesia for its intended, defensive purpose while eliminating as much of the symptom as is practical.

The fact that patients almost always have access to their memories under hypnosis or during barbiturate interview is reassuring to patients and families, and helps establish the diagnosis (MacHovec, 1981; Ruedrich, Chu, & Wadle, 1985). Small amounts of IV amphetamine during barbiturate procedures, to titrate the level of consciousness and allow more verbal interchange, is helpful for some patients.

Conservative Treatment. Another approach, which may be used alone or in combination with the above methods, is that of providing a supportive environment in which the psyche may allow its barriers to be lowered. In some such settings, long, supportive interviews with the patient allow him or her to discuss at length the memories, associations, and feelings that come to mind. In others, the memory returns over a period of days or weeks of support and gentle reminders. Dependency should not be encouraged; brief psychotherapy may be aimed at helping the patient find defenses other than amnesia by which he or she can cope with the emotions and stressful event that precipitated the symptoms.

No matter what method is used, the conflict that precipitated the amnesia should be explored if the patient can tolerate such investigation. One should recall that in this, as well as other neurotic behaviors, the precipitating event is *idiosyncratically* associated with inner conflict, and may not appear particularly stressful to persons other than the patient.

300.60 Depersonalization Disorder (Depersonalization Neurosis)
Nemiah (1980) provides an elegant description of the clinical features of Depersonalization Disorder which are relevant to its treatment and prognosis. He notes that the disorder tends to be chronic, but that many patients experience long periods without symptoms of depersonalization. The association of acute anxiety with onset (or reemergence) of symptoms suggests that many of the treatment approaches for acute

and chronic anxiety (q.v.) may be helpful in the management of symptomatic periods.

Muller (1982) describes successful treatment of acute, severe depersonalization with benzodiazepines. Blue (1979) suggests psychotherapy in which the therapist is quite directive, gaining control of the therapeutic relationship with positive expectations for rapid behavioral change, requiring the patient to think about his or her feelings of depersonalization, and even using paradoxical intention, in which the patient is asked to try to recreate the symptoms.

Barbiturate interviews or hypnosis may provide access to the source of depersonalization symptoms for diagnostic purposes or to provide material for psychotherapy; these acute techniques do not appear to have lasting therapeutic value by themselves.

The patient is usually aware of the dissociative episodes. In those situations in which some *belle indifférence* is present, many clinicians would speak of Briquet's syndrome and apply treatment measures related to those for hysteria (q.v.). In most patients, however, the symptoms are quite frightening.

The depth of psychopathology in persons with severe depersonalization is seen by some as a contraindication to psychoanalytic psychotherapy; however, progress in the analysis of character disorders and disorders of the self should cause the clinician to consider consultation with, or referral to, a qualified psychoanalyst.

Although feelings of "unreality" may sound psychotic, this condition appears clinically and biochemically unrelated to the thought disorders, an observation that is consistent with the lack of success of neuroleptic medication or ECT. Depersonalization sometimes protects against the painful affects of depression. Antidepressant medication may be helpful, but occasionally induces manic psychosis.

300.15 Dissociative Disorder Not Otherwise Specified
Treatment of patients with dissociative symptoms which do not fit any of the above *DSM–III–R* categories should focus upon the symptoms and syndromes as they present, and upon the apparent underlying psychopathology. As implied in the preceding pages, the presence of dissociation suggests a massive defensive effort in the patient. This, in turn, suggests a relatively acute trauma which has rekindled earlier conflicts by virtue of either the strength of the conflicts or the strength of the trauma.

For those patients with relatively good premorbid functioning and/ or well-encapsulated symptoms, a symptomatic approach is likely to be helpful. One example is the treatment of some forms of sleepwalking (somnambulism). Many such patients, after sleepwalking as children, are free of the symptom until some external stress appears in an otherwise uneventful life (e.g., an important loss). Treatment approaches described by Reid (1975; Reid, Ahmed, & Levie, 1981) indicate that symptom removal can occur without psychodynamic complications.

For most dissociative disorders, however, it is important to address both the symptoms and their sources. Dissociative syndromes usually do not lead to serious disability, but return of symptoms at some future time is common.

It is important to recognize the wide variation in total time required for sleep from person to person. Identification of a sleep disorder is therefore largely predicated on the patient's daytime behavior and drowsiness.

SLEEP HYGIENE

All of us have experienced disturbances of the balance between the state of wakefulness and sleep induction systems. Rules for improving the quality of sleep have evolved which can be quite useful to those with transient and milder forms of insomnia. They will not, however, eliminate the more severe forms of sleep disturbance (particularly insomnia). Table 4 provides guidelines for patients who experience minor sleep disturbances.

22A: DYSSOMNIAS

Treatment considerations are predominantly addressed for the chronic or recurring symptom complex. Although the diagnosis often becomes apparent through a detailed history, differentiation of primary vs. secondary insomnia frequently requires polysomnography. Medical consultation may be necessary. Complaints about inadequate sleep are much more significant when the patient also complains of tiredness when awake. To become significant, inadequate sleep should appear at

TABLE 4
Sleep Hygiene

1. Maintain a regular sleep and arousal time.
2. Don't remain in bed after awakening, particularly if you feel rested. Regular morning or afternoon exercise can improve the efficiency of sleep.
3. Avoid warm rooms, which interfere with sleep.
4. Consider a light bedtime snack.
5. Avoid evening caffeine, other stimulants, or alcohol. Nicotine is problematic for many.
6. Mask loud or disturbing noises with an air conditioner, fan, or other source of "white noise." Ear plugs may be helpful.
7. When unable to fall asleep, do not struggle but simply turn on the light, read, write, or even have a light snack until sleepy.

least three times a week for at least one month and remain significant enough to cause daytime fatigue or drowsiness.

INSOMNIA DISORDERS

307.42   Insomnia Disorder Related to Another Mental Disorder (Nonorganic)

This is the most common condition presenting with chronic insomnia. Axis I disorders include depression or other affective disorders, anxiety, and/or adjustment or reactive disorders with anxiety. Many Axis II personality disorders are associated with secondary insomnia. Treatment is directed toward the primary disorder.

In nonpharmacologic management, one must begin with the general sleep hygiene regimen just presented. Kales and Kales (1984) and Coleman and colleagues (1982) have presented excellent recommendations for adjustments in the sleep environment, and in daytime and nighttime activities. Success has been described with behavioral treatments such as biofeedback, stimulus control, relaxation therapy, and the previously mentioned "sleep hygiene."

Spielman, Saskin, and Thorpy (1987) reported sustained improvement in all sleep parameters for up to 36 weeks after a sleep restriction therapy. Extension of an initial marked restriction of time for sleep was based upon improved sleep efficiency. Compliance with this schedule was difficult, but selected patients did achieve satisfactory goals.

At times conjoint marital therapy, particularly when sexual issues are involved, can compliment behavior management. Exercise may be useful, as long as significant exercise activities are avoided near bedtime.

Transient insomnia lends itself quite favorably to pharmacologic management. Inappropriate pharmacologic management can lead to drug abuse. Behavior management is usually more effective in the long run. This is particularly true for the elderly; hypnotic agents should be considered adjuncts to multifaceted treatment. Over-the-counter medications are of no significant assistance in pharmacologic management.

Among the hypnotics, the benzodiazepines have emerged as the primary class of drugs. Roth and colleagues (1982) have demonstrated their effectiveness in reduction of sleep latency, total wake time, and extension of the total sleep time. Benzodiazepines are preferred over barbiturates, antidepressants, antihistamines, and nonbarbiturate sedative-hypnotics. (See Table 5 for a list of benzodiazepines often used to treat insomnia.)

Drug therapy is complicated by side effects such as psychological dependence, drug tolerance, withdrawal symptoms, and daytime hangover. Intermittent use minimizes rebound insomnia, which is particularly common with abrupt discontinuation of the medication. Rebound sleep disorder can be reduced by tapering of the drug (Greenblatt et al., 1987).

In the elderly, diminished metabolism and elimination of all central nervous system depressant drugs prompt one to begin with a minimal dose and to monitor the patient carefully. Many clinicians select compounds with intermediate absorption and elimination rates in order to reach a compromise among daytime sedation, tolerance, and rebound symptoms. Several new benzodiazepines are being studied in this regard (Clark et al., 1986; Dominguez et al., 1986; Rickels et al., 1986).

Chlormethiazole is a rapidly metabolized sedative hypnotic derived from vitamin B1. It has proved to be a popular choice in Europe for treatment of insomnia in elderly patients. In several double-blind studies, published by Bayer and his group, chlormethiazole was as effective as triazolam or temazepam (Bayer et al., 1986; Pathy, Bayer, & Stoker, 1986). Interest in the delta-sleep-inducing peptide (DSIP) remains in experimental stage at this time (Schneider-Helmert, 1986).

L-tryptophan, a precursor of serotonin, is quite popular for the treatment of insomnia. The effective dose is 1–2 gm at bedtime. A recent review suggested that L-tryptophan is effective in both situational

TABLE 5
Benzodiazepines Frequently Used in the Treatment of Insomnia

Drug	Hypnotic Dose (mg)	Absorption Rate	Elimination Rate
Diazepam	5–10	Rapid	Slow
Flurazepam*	15–30	Intermediate	Slow
Triazolam*	0.125–0.5	Intermediate	Rapid
Lorazepam	2–4	Intermediate	Intermediate
Alprazolam	0.25–0.5	Intermediate	Intermediate
Prazepam	10–50	Slow	Slow
Oxazepam	15–30	Slow	Intermediate
Temazepam*	15–30	Slow	Intermediate
Halazepam	20–40	Slow	Slow

* marketed as a hypnotic

and chronic psychophysiologic types of insomnia. Absence of serious side effects and lack of tolerance in long-term trials make it an attractive first-choice prescription (Schneider-Helmert & Spinweber, 1986).

780.50   Insomnia Disorder Related to a Known Organic Factor

This condition addresses 15%–20% of patients with chronic insomnia, and includes conditions that occur only during sleep (e.g., nocturnal myoclonus, restless leg syndrome, sleep apnea, childhood onset insomnia, sleep-related seizure disorders, and nonrestorative sleep).

Among the somatic disorders that commonly lead to insomnia, infectious diseases with high fever, heart disease, hypertension, pulmonary disorders, and gastrointestinal diseases lead the list. Chronic renal insufficiency, endocrine disorders such as hypothyroidism and diabetes, and both acute and chronic states of pain may be associated with insomnia or hyposomnia.

Insomnia secondary to drug use may be the result of bronchodilators, energizing antidepressants, central nervous system stimulants, steroids, and central adrenergic blockers. Adjustments in medication or treatment side effects can prevent most symptoms, without resorting to inappropriate use of hypnotics to counteract these side effects. Benzodiazepine hypnotics with short half-lives can induce insomnia in the latter portion of the night. Caffeinated beverages and cigarette smoking may impair the initiation of sleep. Alcohol will interrupt sleep, inducing difficulty maintaining sleep.

Sleep-related seizure disorders may prove quite difficult to identify but produce symptoms of nocturnal awakening, reducing sleep efficiency. Appropriate diagnostic studies, which include overnight EEG monitoring, may lead to anticonvulsant therapy. Standard polysomnography may not provide adequate EEG channels for proper diagnosis.

Childhood-onset insomnia suggests a developmental, neurochemical imbalance which persists into adulthood and may be accompanied by secondary behavior such as fear of sleep. This condition is frequently associated with learning disabilities and attention deficit disorders. Treatment for those conditions may also alter sleep efficiency. These patients are often quite sensitive to environmental stimulants such as caffeinated beverages. In addition to the standard general recommendations for activity and sleep hygiene adjustments, low doses of amitriptyline (10–50 mg) at bedtime often reduces sleep latency in these patients.

Nonrestorative sleep suggests a difference in the distribution of sleep staging, implying an altered arousal threshold. These patients appear to have adequate total sleep time but continue to complain of daytime malaise and joint aches and pains. L-tryptophan does not appear to be useful; low doses of amitriptyline may relieve the symptoms. Moldofsky and Lue (1980) demonstrated reduction of sleep disturbance and alpha intrusions and improvement in the patient's daytime well-being with chlorpromazine, 100 mg at bedtime.

307.42 Primary Insomnia

After one has eliminated insomnias secondary to psychiatric and medical disorders, 15%–30% of patients (in whom poor sleep patterns represent the only complaint) remain. Total sleep time appears to be within normal limits, but the patient complains of lack of satisfaction with his night's sleep. This group may include naturally short sleepers, subtle sleep-phase syndromes, and individuals with abnormal expectations about sleep. Some are labeled hypochondriacal in spite of psychophysiologic sleep disturbance.

The resolve to obtain a satisfactory night's rest following prolonged stress leads to increased effort which often leads to greater difficulty yet. Such patients often have difficulty returning to efficient sleep after the stress has resolved. This group might benefit from the sleep restriction therapy discussed previously.

Additional therapies which have proved useful include stimulus-control behavior therapy, described by Bootzin and Nicassio (1978). Many can benefit from relaxation therapy and intermittent judicious use of hypnotics. Stress reduction, which must be closely monitored and controlled, is tied to the success of the behavioral techniques.

HYPERSOMNIA DISORDERS

Patients with these disorders experience excessive daytime sleepiness or somnolence despite an adequate night's rest: individuals with one-to-two-hour daytime sleep attacks, excessively prolonged nocturnal sleep, or prolonged transition from the sleeping to fully awake state. Those patients who have a disturbed night's sleep from anxiety, insomnia, or poor health are excluded. The consequences of these symptoms may be devastating to the individual with regard to social impact, employment, underachievement, and impaired school performance.

While studies of excessive daytime somnolence would suggest a prevalence of 0.3%–4% of the adult population (Bixler et al., 1976; Karacan et al., 1976), the percentage of patients presenting to a sleep laboratory is considerably greater. The incidence of treatable medical problems is much higher than in patients complaining of insomnia.

Besides the patient's complaint, the standard approach to measurement of the daytime drowsiness is the Multiple Sleep Latency Test (MSLT) developed by Richardson and colleagues (1978). Sleep latency following the command to fall asleep on five successive occasions is measured every other hour from 10 a.m. A consistent latency of less than 5–10 minutes is abnormal.

307.44   Hypersomnia Disorder Related to Another Mental Disorder (Nonorganic)

This disorder affects about 15% of hypersomnic patients. It is particularly common in the depressive phase of bipolar illness, as well as in dysthymic disorders. It is also common in younger patients with symptoms of depression, schizophrenia, and borderline mental disorders. It is to be distinguished from amnesias and fugue states. One important feature is that the patient awakens unrefreshed even after prolonged sleep. Such individuals may also manifest weight loss, reduced concentration, appetite disturbance and fatigue.

Treatment for this condition is directed toward the primary nonorganic mental disorder. Hypersomnia will often respond to tricyclic antidepressants and monoamine oxidase inhibitors (O'Regan, 1974).

780.50   Hypersomnia Disorder Related to a Known Organic Factor

This disorder affects over 85% of hypersomnic patients, including those with physical conditions, substance abuse, or medication use. Medications that induce these symptoms include hypnotics, tranquilizers, stimulants (rebound from their use), and alcohol. Treatment is dosage adjustment or withdrawal. Withdrawal from caffeine and other stimulants can also be complicated by hypersomnolence.

A second type of hypersomnia is apparent only during sleep: sleep apnea, restless leg syndrome, and narcolepsy. In one series of 283 consecutive patients with daytime drowsiness, 180 were diagnosed with narcolepsy and cataplexy, while only 10 patients were found to have sleep apnea (Parkes, 1981). In the majority of sleep disorders centers, sleep apnea is the most common diagnosis. These primary disorders must be distinguished from hypersomnolence due to medical disorders such as uremia, liver failure, diabetes, hypothyroidism, brain tumors, and anoxic encephalopathies.

Narcolepsy. Treatment of narcolepsy (and frequently accompanying cataplexy or hypnagogic phenomena) must consider its psychosocial and economic impact. The patient may mistakenly be considered psychotic or lazy (Kales et al., 1982). The narcoleptic must adjust his daily activities to his sleep attacks. A nap of 30–60 minutes should be scheduled as needed, after which the narcoleptic symptoms will abate for several hours. These individuals should avoid shift work and occupations involving frequent travel or driving. Their symptoms are exacerbated by drugs with sedative side effects.

Central nervous system stimulant therapy will be required in most cases, most commonly methylphenidate or dextroamphetamine. Guilleminault, Carskadon, and Dement (1974) noted that in a series of 31 patients, dosages greater than 100 mg of dextroamphetamine daily were no more effective than lower doses. In some patients higher doses actually increased daytime drowsiness. Higher doses and long-term therapy are associated with headache, irritability, palpitations, and insomnia. One should try to limit dextroamphetamine to 10–30 mg per day and methylphenidate to 10–40 mg per day. When tolerance appears, the drug should be withdrawn for several weeks or an alternative drug instituted. The danger of medication abuse is obvious.

Pemoline, 40–120 mg per day, is often favored for its longer half-life and once-daily administration. Pemoline has been used for hyperactivity in children with reasonable safety. Phenmetrazine, 25–75 mg daily in up to three divided doses, may be used as an alternative therapy. Since it was introduced in the 1950s for its anorectic affect, phenmetrazine has been noted also to induce mood changes and has a high incidence of misuse (Martin et al., 1971).

The monoamine oxidase inhibitors have not routinely been utilized for this condition, although a recent British report by Roselaar and colleagues (1987) suggests improvement with selegiline, a specific monoamine-oxidase-B inhibitor, in 21 patients. Its effectiveness may be related to its internal conversion to amphetamine. Twenty mg induced subjective improvement in the alert state for four to eight hours. Propranolol in doses of 40–360 mg per day has provided subjective improvement in selected patients (Kales et al., 1979). Finally, gamma-hydroxybutyrate has been demonstrated by several investigators to show promise in the reduction of narcoleptic symptoms (Mamelak & Webster, 1981).

At times, symptoms of cataplexy persist despite the successful treatment of narcolepsy. Tricyclic antidepressants such as clomipramine, 10–100 mg per day, have been described as effective. Some patients develop tolerance (Shapiro, 1975). Clonazepam, 1–4 mg per day, is an alternative.

Menstruation-Associated Hypersomnia. A long-cycle hypersomnia with intervals of sleep prolonged for more than a day has been described with several disorders, including the Kleine-Levine syndrome and a menstruation-linked periodic hypersomnia. Menstruation-associated hypersomnia occurs with a regular and temporal relationship to the menstrual period and is occasionally accompanied by megaphagia. Sleep study often reveals normal nocturnal sleep, but several patients demonstrate paroxysmal EEG discharges (Sachs, Persson, & Hagenfeldt, 1982). Billiard, Guilleminault, and Dement (1975) found that a combination of ethinylestradiol and lynestrenol (oral contraceptives) was successful for many patients.

Kleine-Levine Syndrome. This uncommon disorder involves males with periodic hypersomnia of up to 18–20 hours of sleep per day (recurring monthly to yearly), affective symptoms, and hypothalamic dysfunction. On recovery, the patient may experience total or partial amnesia for his symptoms. Patients appear normal between attacks (Critchley, 1962). Although the condition is considered self-limiting, with recovery occurring in most cases by age 40, Billiard (1981) and others have noted persistence of symptoms for 56 of 96 cases followed for five to nine years. Amphetamines have been reported to reduce both the frequency and severity of the attacks. Lithium carbonate may be an alternative treatment (Goldberg, 1983).

Restless Leg Syndrome. Patients with this condition complain, particularly as they are entering sleep, of an unpleasant, creeping dysesthesia which produces discomfort, weakness and an irresistible need to move the legs (Coleman, 1982). The symptoms have been associated with motor neuron disease, amphetamine use, caffeinism, iron deficiency, anemia, and other metabolic or neoplastic disorders. Patients with restless leg syndrome usually also experience sleep-related myoclonus. When significant arousal occurs during the night, the patient may present with daytime somnolence (Montplaisir et al., 1985).

Treatment is initially directed toward associated medical disorders and deficiencies. Clonidine, up to 0.3mg hs, may bring symptomatic relief (Handwerker & Palmer, 1985). Hening and colleagues (1986) reported relief of restlessness, dysesthesias, dyskinesias while awake, and sleep disturbance following administration of opioids, including propoxyphene, codeine, and methadone.

Sleep Myoclonus. Nocturnal arrhythmic, repetitive twitching is more common than the restless leg syndrome; approximately one-third of patients also have restless legs. Sleep-related myoclonus appears in 12% of insomniacs and 3% of patients with excessive daytime somnolence (Coleman, 1982). The patient is often unaware of the movements yet complains of nonrefreshing sleep. Duration varies from five minutes to several hours during non-REM sleep. Medications, including levo-dopa, tricyclic antidepressants and anticonvulsants, and withdrawal of hypnotic drugs have been associated with the symptoms.

Clonazepam and temazepam have provided symptomatic relief in some patients (Mitler et al., 1986). Guilleminault and Flagg (1984) reported that baclofen decreased the amplitude of the leg movements but not their frequency.

Sleep Apnea. Sleep apnea is found in approximately half of those patients presenting with hypersomnia related to an organic factor. The condition is pathological when more than 30 episodes of 10 seconds or more occur during a single night's sleep, specifically when associated with symptoms of excessive daytime somnolence.

Several types of apnea (central, obstructive, others) can be identified through polysomnography. A number of psychiatric symptoms may develop or be associated with the syndrome, including deterioration in both memory and judgment (particularly during early morning), personality changes, anxiety, and depression. Adults very often have related medical problems, often associated with poor oxygenation of the blood. The diagnosis is confirmed by referral to a sleep laboratory for polysomnographic studies.

Treatment depends upon the severity of the patient's symptoms, oxygen desaturation, and medical status. Milder cases need only avoidance of aggravating medication or substances and/or weight reduction. Avoidance of the supine position for sleep may be effective. In patients with frightening medical sequelae, more aggressive management, beginning with milder surgical procedures, may be necessary.

Treatment should include avoidance of hypnotics, antihistamines, and CNS depressants (including alcohol) before sleep, and may involve a behavior management program. High altitude trips may aggravate problems. Shift work may induce sleep deprivation and aggravate mild sleep apnea. Many patients with chronic obstructive pulmonary disease, appearing as a consequence of sleep apnea and/or contributing to its severity, are made worse by smoking. Steroids may induce obesity and soft tissue hypertrophy, thereby aggravating the obstructive component.

Significant obesity requires the combined approach of diet, stress reduction, and behavior modification. Surgical procedures for weight reduction may be necessary.

In severe conditions, low-flow oxygen therapy (Smith, Haponik, & Bleeker, 1984), nasal CPAP (continuous positive airway pressure) (Guilleminault et al., 1986, 1987), mechanical devices for positioning the jaw or tongue, and various forms of surgery may be indicated.

Drug therapy is often ineffective. Protriptyline has been suggested for increase in the muscle tone of the upper airway and reduction of REM sleep (Brownell et al., 1982; Smith et al., 1983). The effectiveness of this approach remains unclear. The data are inconclusive concerning the effectiveness of medroxyprogesterone acetate (Rajagopal et al., 1986), naloxone, theophylline, acetazolamide, and L-tryptophan.

780.54 Primary Hypersomnia

This condition has no obvious organic cause or relationship to any other disorder. Van den Hoed and colleagues (1981) suggest that this idiopathic disorder represents a neurochemical imbalance. For some patients, there is prolonged nocturnal sleep (12–20 hours) with sleep drunkenness upon awakening, but little refreshed feeling. Symptoms, including sleeping through alarms, often begin in adolescence. This is a non-REM sleep disorder in which approximately one-third of patients have an affected first-degree relative.

Morning doses of stimulants (e.g., dextroamphetamine 10 mg, methylphenidate 20 mg, pemoline 37.5 mg) may be effective. In those patients with almost a 24-hour hypersomnia cycle, a late evening dose may prove useful. Wyler, Wilkins, and Trupin (1975) suggested a trial of methysergide, 2–6 mg per day.

307.45 Sleep-Wake Schedule Disorder

The sleep-wake cycle is directed by a biological, circadian rhythm of approximately 24–28 hours which persists even in a time-free environment. Disorders of sleep schedule can be produced by damage to the suprachiasmic nuclei of the hypothalamus from trauma, infection, degeneration, and/or other disorders (Hauri, 1977). Synchronization or resetting of the biological clock is accomplished through "zeitgebers" which represent time indicators, the most powerful of which is the regular wake-up time. Others include clocks, positions of the sun, work periods, mealtimes, and even low-frequency electromagnetic fields. Medications may lengthen or shorten the circadian rhythms cycle.

There are three types of sleep-wake cycle disorders: the delayed and advanced sleep-phase syndrome, disorganized sleep or irregular sleep-wake patterns, and symptoms that accompany frequently changing sleep-wake times (e.g., from shift work or "jet lag").

Advanced or Delayed Type. Individuals with this disorder experience a shift in their entire sleep process, for example, falling asleep at 3:00 a.m. and awakening seven to eight hours later. The most popular treatment approach is to progressively delay onset of sleep for two to three hours each night until the cycle has been shifted to a more appropriate setting (Weitzman et al., 1981). Following this shift, the individual must strictly adhere to his or her new schedule. There have been several reports of successful treatment of the advanced sleep-phase syndrome by phase-advance chronotherapy moving in the opposite direction (Moldofsky, Musisi, & Phillipson, 1986).

Brief trials of short-acting benzodiazepines have been attempted. Seidel and colleagues found that triazolam, 0.5 mg, modified both the nocturnal insomnia and daytime drowsiness in five patients. Recent studies indicate that exposure to bright light (2,000–2,500 lux) between 8:00 and 10:00 p.m. may be quite effective in treating the advanced sleep-phase syndrome. The delayed sleep-phase syndrome has been shown to respond to bright light exposure in the morning (Lawy, Sack, & Singer, 1985; Lawy et al., 1983).

Disorganized Type. This problem occurs throughout adulthood, more commonly in the older patient who has no set work schedule. It is often self-perpetuating, and requires a gradual reestablishment of the regular day/night cycle, perhaps with mild exercise when the patient becomes drowsy. Daytime naps should be abolished and time in bed should be restricted to those hours designated for sleep. An in-house trainer or even hospitalization may be needed to reestablish a regular cycle. Weekends are particularly dangerous for return to old habits.

Symptoms Due to Frequent Changes in Sleep/Wake Times. Occasionally, individuals (for example, "on-call" workers, international travellers) will attempt to alter these symptoms with stimulants or sedative-forced sleep. Individuals with a permanent night shift have difficulty establishing a consolidated sleep period. Previously efficient sleepers fare better with work shifts and night shift responsibilities than do persons with histories of sleep problems. Transient use of bedtime short-acting benzodiazepines can be tried, if the patient's schedule change is permanent, to establish the new sleep/wake cycle. In severe cases, the patient may have to change jobs (Afchoff, Hoffman, & Pohl, 1975).

307.40 Dyssomnia Not Otherwise Specified

Complete discussion of all other dyssomnias is not possible. The clinician may consider the principles just outlined, and should make use of referral resources in other specialties as appropriate.

22B: PARASOMNIAS

307.47 Dream Anxiety Disorder (Nightmare Disorder)

Nightmares or dream anxiety episodes frequently do not contain the screams nor the excessive autonomic symptoms noted in night terrors. Instead, the patient manifests a motor component with rolling or thrashing about in the bed, but upon awakening is able to recall the dream and present a clear sensorium. These events occur predominantly out of REM sleep in the middle and latter parts of the night. Patients experiencing a Post-traumatic Stress Disorder may manifest a striking imagery during the drowsy state between wakefulness and sleep.

These symptoms are frequently transient, particularly in the younger age groups, and require only temporary psychiatric support or benzodiazepine hypnotic. It is important to recall that nightmares may be associated with drug treatment withdrawal.

307.46 Sleep Terror Disorder

Among the parasomnias, night terrors evoke the most concern from the patient. These episodes are characterized by extreme terror and panic, often punctuated by a piercing cry. They are associated with autonomic discharges such as tachycardia, sweating, mydriasis, and hypertension. These events are distinguished from nightmares because they are not followed by a full degree of alertness with clear sensorium. Sleep terrors occur 60–90 minutes after sleep onset.

They are relatively more common in children; adult presentation is often associated with psychopathology. Many patients demonstrate inhibition of aggression. Obsessive-compulsive tendencies and phobias accompanied by both anxiety and depression are common accompanying features which should be thoroughly investigated by the clinician.

Psychotherapy may be appropriate following the diagnostic evaluation. Suppression of Stage III/IV sleep with benzodiazepines or other carefully chosen hypnotics may prove useful, although many hypnotics increase Stage III/IV sleep time and thus may worsen symptoms.

Imipramine has also been used. Medication is rarely required for this condition in children.

307.46 Sleepwalking Disorder

Somnambulism or sleepwalking manifests as an automatism which varies from sitting up in bed to leaving one's bed and walking about in a confused part-waking, part-sleeping state. Most episodes last only a few seconds or minutes, with occasional recall of the events upon awakening. The risk of injury mandates adjustments in the patient's environment similar to those mentioned above for sleep terrors.

In children, sleepwalking is generally benign and rarely requires therapy. There is very often a family history of similar symptoms. In adults, the appearance of symptoms is often associated with unusual tension or stress in a person with a childhood history of sleepwalking. The clinician must identify any psychopathology or neurologic disease and initiate appropriate measures. There is frequently no diagnosable mental or physical illness.

The management of patients with sleepwalking requires stringent safety measures to prevent the patient from accidental injury. This may mean special locks for the doors and windows as well as sleeping on the ground floor. The old adage about precipitating violent behavior if one interrupts sleepwalking is largely myth, although awakening should be gentle and confusion should be expected.

Reid (1975) demonstrated sustained effect of six hypnotherapy sessions in young adults with uncomplicated, intractable sleepwalking, using specialized conditioning to tactile cues. Low doses of diazepam (5–10 mg at bedtime) have worked for similar patients (Reid, Ahmed, and Levie, 1981). Tolerance is not a problem, as the effect appears to be related to regulation of sleep cycles rather than alleviation of anxiety. Imipramine, 10–50 mg at bedtime, has also been reported to be of use, particularly in children with intractable symptoms and/or combinations of parasomnias.

In the elderly, one should consider low doses of neuroleptics (e.g., haloperidol 0.5 mg) rather than the benzodiazepines. Geriatric symptoms are often associated with an organic brain syndrome.

307.40 Parasomnia Not Otherwise Specified

The motor parasomnias include restless leg syndrome or periodic repetitive myoclonic-like leg movements (particularly occurring as the patient enters sleep). The benzodiazepines—particularly clonazepam 1–3 mg hs or hypnotic doses of temazepam—remain the accepted treatment for such disorders. Clonidine may also be effective (cf., its use in Tourette's Disorder).

Nocturnal head-banging or body-rocking, sometimes seen in adolescents or adults following head injury, may respond to imipramine.

Other parasomnias should be carefully evaluated and treated according to their symptoms and the principles already discussed. Referral to a neurologist or other sleep disorders subspecialist is often indicated.

Patients who are particularly vengeful or who have been severely exploited or abused are relatively poorer candidates (Silver, 1983; Stone, 1985b). Uncontrolled substance abuse and paraphilias traditionally predict poor response. Intractable acting-out renders the patient unavailable for outpatient therapy. Some of these relative contraindications can be circumvented if the patient can be treated in a long-term residential setting.

Stone (1987) stresses that one of the most important transactions in reconstructive therapy involves the therapist's ability to recognize his own reactions, to understand the source of his countertransference within the patient's psyche, and to translate this understanding for the patient. This important use of countertransference brings out feelings (especially angry ones) which the patient has, but disowns.

The treatment itself includes strong relationships between patient and therapist, within which the patient can move as needed from extreme closeness to considerable distance, but which encourages separation-individuation and tolerance for therapeutic interventions (Horwitz, 1985). Early in the work, content deserves more active attention than process, and negative feelings toward the therapist-object should be made as conscious as possible (Waldinger, 1987). Throughout treatment, the therapist will need to insert support and "real" intervention, often followed by observation or interpretation of the situation which gave rise to the need for such actions.

There are many controversies within the literature and among clinicians with regard to proper therapeutic stance, the order of addressing various psychodynamic issues, tolerance for various behaviors of the patient, and the like. The reader is referred to references cited for further discussion.

Diagnostic continua or spectra, particularly between Borderline and Narcissistic Personality Disorders and between character pathology and neurosis, have suggested that many borderline patients who are successful in psychotherapy or psychoanalysis begin to look increasingly narcissistic. This is considered by Adler (1980) to be a goal of treatment for such patients, and the antithesis of retreat into schizoid isolation.

The treatment of Narcissistic Personality Disorder (q.v.) is often discussed with, and compared to, the treatment of Borderline Personality Disorder. Adler (1986) agrees with most other clinicians that the first few months of psychotherapy consist largely of support and empathy, early clarification of countertransference, and awareness of the power of the patient's issues of anger and aloneness. Success in this phase leads to attempts at optimal frustration within the psychotherapy, and the experiencing of self-object transferences with the therapist.

In spite of the extensive literature and interesting discussion among clinicians about the psychotherapeutic treatment of Borderline Personality Disorder, there remains little in the way of nonanecdotal description of treatment techniques to guide the psychotherapist (Frosch, 1983). In Silver's words (1983), such treatment may still be considered "therapeutic heroics."

Group Therapy. A wide variety of group therapy experiences may be helpful for borderline patients. Some are practical and related to day-to-day issues, such as parenting skills and experiences groups (Holman, 1985). Others are quite intensive, offering consistent, analytically oriented environments for reality testing, growth, and change (Kretsch, Goren, & Wasserman, 1987; Macaskill, 1982). The importance of group involvement in long-term inpatient settings, both as a part of a therapeutic community and as a vehicle for internal exploration, has already been addressed.

Medications. Unlike the case with some other personality disorders, judicious choice of medication can affect the course of Borderline Personality Disorder. On the other hand, like hysteroid and schizotypal patients, the borderline individual is often inordinately sensitive to side effects, poorly compliant, and exhibits capricious-appearing vacillations of symptoms—even metamorphoses—that are distressing to the ordered style of many biological psychiatrists.

Antipsychotic medications are the ones most often considered, and may be prescribed either for the occasional acute psychosis seen in these patients or for their chronic (especially schizotypal) symptoms. For acute psychosis, routine doses of high-potency neuroleptics such as thiothixene or haloperidol are used (see Chapter 14).

Schizotypal symptoms (i.e., near-psychotic eccentricities and anxieties) are the next most frequently considered indication. Low doses are sufficient. Thiothixene in the general range of 6–12 mg per day is sometimes found to be superior to haloperidol; however, both appear to address cognitive disturbance, derealization, ideas of reference, anxiety, and even depression in borderline patients (see below) (Goldberg et al., 1986; Serban & Siegel, 1984). Addition of adjunctive drugs has not been well studied. An understanding of the psychodynamic meaning of medication, particularly in patients engaged in psychotherapy, should include considering pills as transitional objects (Adelman, 1985).

The use of antidepressants in Borderline Personality is often disappointing. At least one series of double-blind comparisons indicated uniformly better results from neuroleptics than from tricyclic antidepressants in reducing overall symptom severity (Soloff et al., 1986a,b). Cole and colleagues (1984), however, found that tricyclics were effective for borderline patients with specific symptoms of major depression. These studies reflect the general clinical feeling that severe depressive symptoms in borderline patients should be treated with antidepressants, in spite of a relative dearth of research support. There is at least one report of severe adverse reactions to tricyclic antidepressants in borderline patients, including increased suicide threats, assaultive behavior, and paranoid ideation (Soloff, 1986c).

Many other medications may be prescribed for specific symptoms or syndromes, although the response in borderline patients may not be as good as that expected in patients with uncomplicated Axis I disorders. Thus, patients with hypomanic symptoms may respond to lithium, some depressed or primitively self-destructive patients to MAO inhibitors, and so forth. Gardner and Cowdry (1986) reported some decrease in behavioral dyscontrol when carbamazepine was prescribed for borderline women with intractable impulsiveness.

Medication should never been given without adequate psychosocial intervention. Repeated use of medication for patients' frequent complaints of anxiety may sometimes be necessary, but should be viewed with caution.

Outcome and Follow-up. Many of the indicators for psychotherapeutic or psychoanalytic success discussed above are associated with relatively better outcome for the patient, and sometimes a good prognosis. Woollcott (1985) proposes a similar list of prognostic indicators for psychotherapy. Waldinger and Gunderson (1984) examined the outcome of 78 borderline patients of some 11 experienced psychotherapists. They came to the general conclusion that the longer patients stayed in treatment, the more they improved. In addition, the more prior treatment the patient had, the better the therapeutic outcome.

This finding is particularly important, since many patients stop therapy prematurely and both patient and therapist may be pessimistic about the future. Subsequent psychotherapy often builds upon the last experience, when the patient is ready for another "step" in his or her growth. Many of the patients in the Waldinger and Gunderson study did not complete treatment, but had made considerable gains in ego function, behavior, object relatedness, and sense of self.

Stone (1987) traced a large number of borderline patients 10 to 23 years after referral for psychoanalytic psychotherapy. He reported that 40% showed "clinical recovery," often after five to 10 years of treatment. Two-thirds had at least a "good" outcome. It may be noted that these patients were treated by very experienced psychotherapists.

301.50   Histrionic Personality Disorder

According to *DSM-III-R*, Histrionic Personality Disorder is identical to "hysterical personality." Kernberg (1986b), however, differentiates the two in a recent psychiatry textbook. To make matters more confusing, psychiatry and the public have various definitions of "hysterical," which are nicely differentiated by Chodoff (1982). For purposes of this chapter, we will refer to patients who meet *DSM-III-R* criteria for Histrionic Personality Disorder and to symptoms they are likely to present.

Although medications may be indicated for acute psychotic or depressive symptoms, most superficial and characterologic symptoms are best addressed with psychotherapy. Hysterical neurosis should be differentiated from hysterical or Histrionic Personality, the personality disorder being considerably more complicated to treat. Sometimes this differentiation cannot be made until the patient has revealed the character pathology in several weeks or months of psychoanalytically oriented psychotherapy.

Specific topics to be addressed, or which present particular problems in therapy, cannot be comprehensively addressed in this text, but include early, stormy, and intense transference with erotic-seeming (but not truly erotic) defenses guarding against awareness of great dependency. Patients are often quite seductive, in the sense that they appear to be working on important therapeutic issues and forming positive transferences, while becoming angry at the therapist's lack of total, giving presence. The therapist's skill at knowing when to give and when to judiciously frustrate the patient is critically important.

Kernberg (1986b) feels that Histrionic Personality is likely to worsen without psychotherapy, while hysterical personality may gradually improve as the patient adjusts with age. He suggests prompt treatment, even if severe pathology, intractable acting-out, or antisocial features limit the therapist's interventions to support and superficial exploration.

The therapist should be aware that the reactive aspects of the disorder often lead to anxious, depressive, or other overreactions to minor emotional or external events. Brief counseling techniques should thus be available, even for the patient engaged in ongoing psycho-therapy. Dramatic, impulsive, often poorly-thought-out suicidal behavior is frequently seen. Although it may accurately be interpreted as ma-nipulative or "gesture," such behavior must always be taken seriously, particularly if one is not familiar with the patient. For those with whom the therapist is quite familiar, the principles of availability, consistency, and firmness outlined in the section on Borderline Personality Disorder may be helpful.

301.81 Narcissistic Personality Disorder

The "spectrum" of narcissistic disorders to which Adler (1986) refers has been touched upon in earlier sections of this chapter. Here, we will refer to the many levels at which the patient may have problems with narcissistic needs and expectations, and the accompanying levels of adaptation found (from severe impairment to great social success). The goals of restructuring therapies are increased empathy for others and toward the self; decreased regression in the face of rebuff, failure, or separation; a capacity for flexible detachment and distancing oneself; the ability to feel gratified when working alone; the ability to give without personal gain; and the capacity to truly mourn an important loss (Nurnberg, 1984).

One of the issues in the psychotherapeutic treatment of the suc-cessful narcissistic patient is whether or not he or she has a personality disorder. Ledermann (1982) points out the danger of underdiagnosing these patients, and then discusses their psychoanalysis in much the same way as that of other serious personality disorders. The patient eventually becomes able to integrate his disowned or split-off impulses, experience them as not absolute, and tolerate a world in which love and hate, black and white, can coexist.

Battegay (1985) recognizes a need for a modified psychoanalytic approach, however, in which empathy is important during periods of depression. Ganzarain (1982) discusses opportunities that may be avail-able in group, as opposed to individual, psychotherapy which help the patient consider overcoming his grandiose wish to be his own provider, depending upon no one.

The understanding, and eventual interpretation and working-through, of the grandiose self is the primary task of psychoanalytically oriented treatment. This is often seen in the transference, in which the "real" aspects of the therapeutic relationship are missing and the patient seems emotionally unavailable (Kernberg, 1986a).

The concept of mourning is important to change in narcissistic patients. Protection against significant loss, of real objects, is the major purpose of narcissistic character structure. Warnes (1984) describes a poignant termination phase in which the activation of profound mourning led to structural change.

Nonintensive Treatment. Treatment of reactive or superficial symptoms should progress largely upon the lines discussed for the Axis I disorders and symptoms, with an understanding of the underlying personality disorder. Symptom fluctuations and suicide dangers are of less concern than with Borderline Personality Disorder. The hiding of the patient's pathology through normal-appearing narcissistic defenses and behavior is common; however, the purpose of short-term or crisis treatment is the shoring up of existing defenses, not the restructuring of narcissistic character.

27C: CLUSTER C

301.82 Avoidant Personality Disorder
There have been no research reports of treatment of this disorder since its inclusion in the original *DSM–III*. A few authors suggest differences between the avoidant patient and the schizoid patient (the latter possessing a deficit in relating ability, rather than a defense against relating) or the borderline patient; however, most clinical recommendations are similar to those for Schizoid Personality Disorder.

Most patients never come to treatment because of the security of their "neurotic equilibrium," which would be upset by any change in symptoms. For those who do, initial supportive care and enhancement of self-image may allow some tentative exploration of interactions with others and with the environment within the safety of the therapeutic relationship.

Group therapy offers opportunities to explore growth within a protected setting. A number of behavioral treatments (e.g., desensitization) offer the patient control over progress and change. In addition, specific treatments for symptoms or signs of Axis I disorders such as anxiety or phobia should prove useful, while allowing the patient to retain ego-syntonic avoidance defenses. Psychoanalytically oriented techniques such as those earlier described for the personality disorders probably represent the treatment of choice for a few patients.

301.60 Dependent Personality Disorder

As with many of the other personality disorders, patients with this diagnosis are unlikely to seek treatment. They may, however, wish to explore reasons for lack of social or vocational success, and may suffer considerable loss when an important figure leaves them in one way or another. Referrals of dependent patients within a consultation-liaison framework are common; however, many of these patients' characteristics are related to a medical illness within a hospital setting and do not fill *DSM-III-R* criteria for Dependent Personality Disorder.

The primary therapeutic modality is psychotherapy. Early in therapy, the clinician should accept much of the same dependence that the patient feels toward others in his or her life. Symptoms and psychodynamics can then be discussed firsthand, rather than as reports of feelings about others. The therapist's support of the patient's individuation from others (and now from the therapist as well) should include practical issues such as jobs and housing.

Failure of the highly gratifying dependent style may give rise to anxiety, depression, or other symptoms. These may be superficially treated using suggestions given elsewhere in this book; however, caution should be exercised when considering medication. Anxiolytics are likely to be abused, and antidepressants are inappropriate for reactive symptoms such as these. Behavioral interventions or practical, directive counseling approaches are more likely to help, and less likely to add to the patient's problems in the long run.

One should, however, take these reactive symptoms seriously, since severely dependent patients harbor a potential for overwhelming despondency or rage against the self or others (Kiev, 1976). Profound loss or intense affect in these patients should lead the therapist to consider protective measures such as hospitalization, with which the patient can be contained to some extent and definitive therapy for Axis I symptoms carried out in a controlled setting.

Termination of individual or group psychotherapy is a delicate task, and should be a joint decision. The therapist should be flexible, allowing the patient to return as needed, within reason. Frustration of lingering dependent needs, which one might consider in other kinds of patients to be a therapeutic motivating factor, may have countertherapeutic effects (Malinow, 1981).

301.40 Obsessive Compulsive Personality Disorder

Patients with Obsessive Compulsive Personality Disorder who seek treatment usually do so because the usefulness of this usually effective character style has been compromised. Common symptoms are those of Axis I diagnoses of Obsessive Compulsive Disorder, Affective Disorder, or occasionally Paranoia. The patient is often quite anxious, and motivated for psychotherapy. The short-term treatments for Obsessive Compulsive Disorder described elsewhere in this text are often effective. Behavioral and psychotherapeutic treatments for depression or anxiety, or anxiolytic medication, are usually effective. Reconstitution of the previously effective personality disorder usually preempts any need for tricyclic antidepressants or longer-term care.

For motivated patients, the definitive treatment is insight-oriented or psychoanalytic psychotherapy. Needs for control and related fears of destructive impulses are important issues at all levels of treatment, from simple scheduling requests, to intellectualization and rationalization, to other resistances against fantasy and free association. Many of the characteristics that lead to a successful life for such a patient and that appear to the inexperienced therapist to create an excellent therapy candidate are actually symptoms that can become serious impediments to treatment (Tarachow, 1963).

The therapist must avoid competing with the patient and should be able to tolerate his verbal attacks, retaining a therapeutic posture rather than allowing sessions to deteriorate into intellectual discussions or nonproductive interchange. Patients who show signs of deteriorating should probably be treated less intensively and more actively. In some cases, cognitive therapy may be tried (Quality Assurance Project, 1985). Although many patients will have read a psychiatry text and may request specific medications or therapies, the clinician's treatment decisions should be continued, and the patient's behavior observed or interpreted as resistance.

301.84 Passive Aggressive Personality Disorder

Treatment of these patients is similar to, but may be less rewarding than, the treatment of the patient with Dependent Personality Disorder. Psychotherapy is likely to be frustrating; however, the fact that the passive-aggressive symptoms often severely interfere with work or social goals may motivate the patient to participate long enough to form a therapeutic alliance. Clear rules of therapy must be outlined; those that involve schedules, billing, and the like should be provided in writing. This prevents spending inordinate amounts of time arguing over something that the patient calls forgetfulness, but the therapist calls (sometimes pejoratively) resistance. Passive-aggressive patients respond to the therapist much as they respond to others in their lives, whom they often perceive to be unfairly demanding.

Presenting symptoms of either failure of the passive-aggressive coping style or problems with the patient's environment guide initial interventions toward Axis I-like symptoms, usually of anxiety or depression. Although it is tempting to use their distress as fuel for commitment to psychotherapy, patients who cannot escape their defensive binds or environmental situations through their usual passive-aggressive resources may escalate their defensive behavior, even to the point of suicide attempts. When possible, one should not confuse passive-aggressive sources of self-destructive behavior with major affective disorder, and should avoid antidepressants. Protective hospitalization is occasionally required; the patient has now thrown down a gauntlet of confrontation or panic, which the therapist should not firmly challenge.

In this and other treatment situations, countertransference and related issues must be carefully considered. One commonly hears the term "passive-aggressive" used to connote manipulative or frustrating patients in a way that is punishing or derisive. Although the clinician may feel angry, he or she should be flexible and remember that the patient's behavior, even if apparently voluntary, is defending against severe anxiety or deterioration. On the other hand, if the therapist's "giving in" is seen as ambivalence or abandoning of therapeutic interest, the patient may feel bereft and the therapeutic alliance may be injured.

Directive and behavioral techniques, such as assertiveness training, offer concrete ways to address the patient (Perry & Flannery, 1982). These should be considered symptomatic treatment, however, except when added to a comprehensive plan for long-term psychotherapy.

301.90 Personality Disorder Not Otherwise Specified
Patients who qualify for this residual category should be treated based upon the clinician's estimate of presenting symptoms, personality dynamics, and developmental level, and interactions among them.

Chapter 28

V Codes for Conditions Not Attributable to a Mental Disorder That Are a Focus of Attention or Treatment

V62.30 Academic Problem

Treatment of this disorder in the absence of any other diagnosable mental disorder should be based upon simple counseling with exploration of possible family or environmental stresses. As with many of the other V Code conditions, one should be aware of the dangers of overdiagnosis and mislabeling of conditions not attributable to a mental disorder.

V71.01 Adult Antisocial Behavior

Few treatment approaches are effective for repeated antisocial behavior which is not due to one of the mental disorders already discussed (including a reactive Adjustment Disorder). Individual and group psychotherapy alone have poor records of success, as do all of the biological therapies, ordinary psychiatric hospitalization, or simple incarceration.

Inpatient hospitalization at institutions such as those discussed under Antisocial Personality Disorder may be successful for some patients; however, the majority of patients with adult antisocial behavior do not commit crimes sufficient to allow their being sentenced to several years of maximum security treatment. For many of these people, the community and wilderness treatment programs discussed under Antisocial Personality Disorder have met with some success and are quite cost-effective (Cytrynbaum & Ken, 1975; Kimball, 1979; Reid & Matthews, 1980; Reid & Solomon, 1981).

V40.00　Borderline Intellectual Functioning

This category, which is made up of the majority of individuals society calls "mentally retarded," does not represent true mental retardation (Strider & Menolascino, 1981). For the most part, these people have few serious difficulties in society; however, they may be prone to problems in those areas in which one's cognitive abilities or fund of knowledge are important for coping with personal or environmental problems. Supportive treatment, along with relevant education for the patient when such problems or crises develop, is almost always helpful. One may wish to counsel the family as well and to be sure that the patient knows of available help from social agencies (e.g., employment counseling for a worker who has lost his job).

Much of the frustration of the person with Borderline Intellectual Functioning is related to how he or she is treated by an uninformed or prejudiced public. Discussions with community, school, or work officials may be helpful. When problems are more troublesome (as in a person with an accompanying Conduct Disorder), flexible, practical therapeutic measures should be employed rather than traditional approaches such as individual or group psychotherapy (although some group therapy is highly effective). Institutionalization or other infantilizing procedures are never necessary for the treatment of Borderline Intellectual Functioning per se.

V71.02　Childhood or Adolescent Antisocial Behavior

The treatment of many of these behaviors is discussed earlier in the text, in both the section on Disorders Usually First Evident in Infancy, Childhood, or Adolescence and the section on Antisocial Personality Disorder (although persons of this age should never be given the diagnosis of Antisocial Personality Disorder). It is important that children or adolescents not be given this diagnosis if their antisocial behavior forms a pattern that can be diagnosed elsewhere in the *DSM-III-R*.

Unfortunately, it has become common for children or adolescents with simple antisocial behavior to be placed in psychiatric hospitals. In some cases, this is because of well-meaning parents, judges, or probation officers who feel that psychiatric hospitalization is preferable to juvenile detention or jail. In others, it seems related to the marketing of adolescent hospital beds by enthusiastic providers. In either case, adding an indelible record of psychiatric hospitalization and fostering a "sick" self-image is rarely helpful in the long run. In addition, the brief hospitalization usually available in acute-care hospitals does not adequately address many kinds of delinquency. Specialized programs for conduct disorders may be effective.

V65.20 Malingering
Since by definition there is no primary illness to treat once malingering has been established, there remain only a couple of issues of management of the patient who is felt to be voluntarily misrepresenting his or her symptoms for some conscious reason not associated with factitious illness (e.g., to obtain money, avoid work, or avoid responsibility for criminal behavior). The most obvious of these is to offer understanding and counsel to the person who feels that he or she must use this dishonest course of action. Education with respect to social agencies available to help with financial problems, the possible consequences of one's dishonesty, or even the fact that faking an illness really *is* dishonest, and a serious misuse of resources may be beneficial.

The temptation to tell someone about the malingering should be resisted. In addition to the possibility that the patient is not malingering, this author would disagree with Getto (1982) that one of the treatment goals is to make the malingering "diagnosis" available to legal, health, and social agencies with which the patient may have contact. The physician who does this runs considerable risk of breach of ethics and could under some circumstances be liable for slander or libel. It seems more prudent, if less gratifying, to note in the record that one is unable to find any medical or psychological basis for the individual's complaints.

V61.10 Marital Problem
In the absence of other mental disorder, including Adjustment Disorder, the goals of the therapist are generally to provide information and counseling, be an objective observer, recognize problems in communication and facilitate their resolution, and avoid overdiagnosis. To some extent, the therapist may wish to become a negotiator; however, most authors recommend against placing oneself in the position of "referee."

The question of whether a therapist should assist with the completion of a separation or divorce, when he or she feels that it is appropriate or inevitable, may arise. The clinician should be certain that such decisions are made by one or both members of the couple, and not by the therapist, before proceeding. Although patients may describe symptoms that make the diagnosis of Axis I disorders tempting, in themselves or in their partners, marital problems in their normal course should be treated without extensive diagnosis or overtreatment.

Some therapists treat both husband and wife individually, or provide both conjoint and individual counseling. This approach is usually ill-advised and fraught with opportunities for misunderstanding and conflict of interest. An additional therapist should be chosen for each person if individual work is needed.

V15.81 Noncompliance with Medical Treatment
Noncompliance in the absence of any of the mental disorders already described may be treated with education (about one's illness or the treatment involved) or counseling. Since the patient generally has a right not to comply (except in some narrowly circumscribed legal situations), counseling with family members or with frustrated medical staff who are having difficulty accepting the patient's decision may be indirectly helpful. For example, a clinician may ease tensions between nursing staff and the patient which might adversely affect other aspects of the patient's care.

V62.20 Occupational Problems
The same basic treatment principles apply as were mentioned above under Academic Problem (V62.30). One may also wish to consider some of the issues discussed in the chapter on Adjustment Disorders.

V61.20 Parent–Child Problem
The general principles of counseling in parent-child problems are occasionally similar to those of marital problems; however, practical issues, psychodynamics, and the fact that one member of the parent-child dyad is a child make specific issues quite different. The variety of potential conflicts and problems that may arise and the intricacy of family therapies involved make complete discussion impossible in this section. Helpful information may be found in the section on Disorders Usually First Evident in Infancy, Childhood, or Adolescence, and in other texts. Specific training and experience in child psychiatry are recommended.

V62.81 Other Interpersonal Problems
These conditions should be addressed according to the presenting complaints and situations as perceived by the clinician. General principles of education, counseling, and avoidance of overdiagnosis apply.

V61.80 Other Specified Family Circumstances

These conditions should be addressed according to the presenting complaints and situations as perceived by the clinician. General principles of education, counseling, and avoidance of overdiagnosis apply.

V62.89 Phase of Life Problem or Other Life Circumstance Problem

The tremendous variety of problems that might fall into this category is too broad to address completely. The educational and counseling principles already discussed should suffice for most cases. The therapist should be alert for countertransference and related issues; for example, those of a young therapist treating an older patient with concerns about retirement, or a therapist with particular values who attempts to give objective counseling to a patient with opposing views.

V62.82 Uncomplicated Bereavement

The psychiatrist (or more frequently the family physician) may be consulted about some of the more striking symptoms of normal grief. One pitfall of treatment is overdiagnosis. The patient should not be told, or treated as if, he has an aberrant grief reaction or serious depression unless he does not qualify for this V Code condition. Support and guidance may be given, however, with reassurance that the feelings are normal and should not be avoided. The therapist should show approval of the many feelings experienced by the grieving person, including anger for the lost object.

Counseling for the individual and for well-meaning family or friends should include a caveat against overprotection. That is, such activities as attending funeral and memorial services, returning to the home where the deceased lived, and putting away his or her possessions (and, with them, memories) should be encouraged for grieving individuals of all ages. The clinician should make it clear that he or she is available, but need not be intrusive.

Treatment for aberrant or unresolved grief, with persistent yearning, overidentification with the deceased, and/or inability to express sadness or rage, is addressed in the chapter on Adjustment Disorders.

References for Section IV

Abel, G. G., Becker, J. V., Cunningham-Rather, J., et al.: *The Treatment of Child Molesters.* Behavioral Medicine Laboratory, P. O. Box AF, Emory University, Atlanta, Georgia, 30322. Published 1984.

Achte, K., Lonnqvist, J., Kuusi, K., et al.: Outcome studies on schizophrenic psychoses in Helsinki. *Psychopathology,* 19(1–2):60–67, 1986.

Adelman, S. A.: Pills as transitional objects: A dynamic understanding of the use of medication in psychotherapy. *Psychiatry,* 48(3):246–253, 1985.

Adler, G.: A treatment framework for adult patients with borderline and narcissistic personality disorders. *Bulletin of the Menninger Clinic,* 44(2):171–180, 1980.

Adler, G.: Psychotherapy of the narcissistic personality disorder patient: Two contrasting approaches. *American Journal of Psychiatry,* 143(4):430–436, 1986.

Afchoff, J., Hoffman, K., & Pohl, H.: Re-entrainment of circadian rhythms after phase-shifts of the zeitgeber. *Chronobiologia,* 2(2):23–78, 1975.

Akiskal, H. S., Arana, G. W., Baldessarini, R. J., et al.: A clinical report of thymoleptic-responsive atypical paranoid psychoses. *American Journal of Psychiatry,* 140(9):1187–1190, 1983.

Alexander, F. G.: *Psychosomatic Medicine: Its Principles and Applications.* New York: Norton, 1950.

Alexander, P. E., & Alexander, D. D.: Alprazolam treatment for panic disorders. *Journal of Clinical Psychiatry,* 47(6):301–304, 1986.

Allen, J. G., Colson, D. B., Coyne, L., et al.: Problems to anticipate in treating difficult patients in a long-term psychiatric hospital. *Psychiatry,* 49(4):350–358, 1986.

Allen, C. B., Davis, B. M., & Davis, K. L.: Psychoendocrinology in clinical psychiatry. In R. E. Hales & A. J. Frances (Eds.), *Psychiatry Update, Annual Review, Volume 6.* Washington, D.C.: American Psychiatric Press, 1987, p. 198.

Allsopp, L. F., Huitson, A., Deering, R. B., et al.: Efficacy and tolerability of sustained-release clomipramine (Anafranil SR) in the treatment of phobias: A comparison with the conventional formulation of clomipramine (Anafranil). *Journal of Internal Medicine Research,* 13(4):203–208, 1985.

American Psychiatric Association: *Task Force Report #14: Electroconvulsive Therapy* (F. Frankel [Chairperson] et al.). Washington, D.C.: APA Board of Trustees, 1979.

American Psychiatric Association: *Diagnostic and Statistical Manual of Mental Disorders, Third Edition-Revised.* Washington, D.C.: American Psychiatric Press, 1987.

Ames, D., Burrows, G., Davies, B., et al.: A study of the dexamethasone suppression test in hospitalized depressed patients. *British Journal of Psychiatry*, 144:311–313, 1984.

Ananth, J.: Clomipramine: An antiobsessive drug. *Canadian Journal of Psychiatry*, 31(3):253–258, 1986.

Andrews, E., Bellard, J., & Walter-Ryan, W. G.: Monosymptomatic hypochondriacal psychosis manifesting as delusions of infestation: Case studies of treatment with haloperidol. *Journal of Clinical Psychiatry*, 47(4):188–190, 1986.

Ansseau, M., Doumont, A., Thiry, D., von Frenckell, R., et al.: Initial study of methyl-clonazepam in generalized anxiety disorder. Evidence for greater power in the crossover design. *Psychopharmacology* (Berlin), 87(2):130–135, 1985.

Appel, G.: An approach to the treatment of schizoid phenomena. *Psychoanalytic Review*, 61:99–113, 1974.

Arieti, S.: Psychotherapy of schizophrenia: New or revised procedures. *American Journal of Psychotherapy*, 34(4):464–476, 1980.

Astrup, C.: Querulent paranoia: A follow-up. *Neuropsychobiology*, 11(3):149–154, 1984.

Babiker, I. E.: Comparative efficacy of long-acting depot and oral neuroleptic medications in preventing schizophrenic recidivism. *Journal of Clinical Psychiatry*, 48(3):94–97, 1987.

Baizerman, M., & Emshoff, B.: Juvenile firesetting: Building a community-based prevention program. *Children Today*, 13(3):7–12, 1984.

Ban, T. A., Guy, W., & Wilson, W. H.: The psychopharmacological treatment of depression in the medically ill patient. *Canadian Journal of Psychiatry*, 29(6):461–466, 1984.

Bancroft, J., Davidson, D. W., Warner, T., et al.: Androgens and sexual behaviour in women using oral contraceptives. *Clinical Endocrinology* (Oxford), 12(4):327–340, 1980.

Bancroft, J., O'Carroll, R., McNeilly, A., et al.: The effects of bromocriptine on the sexual behaviour of hyperprolactinaemic men: A controlled case study. *Clinical Endocrinology* (Oxford), 21(2):131–137, 1984.

Bastani, J. B., & Kentsmith, D. K.: Psychotherapy with wives of sexual deviants. *American Journal of Psychotherapy*, 34(1):20–25, 1980.

Battegay, R.: The different narcissistic disturbances of personality and their psychotherapeutic approach. *Psychotherapy and Psychosomatics*, 44(1):46–53, 1985.

Baum, N.: Treatment of impotence. 1. Non-surgical methods. *Postgraduate Medicine*, 81(7):133–136, 1987.

Bayer, A. J., Bayer, E. M., Pathy, M. S. J., et al.: Double-blind controlled study of chlormethiazole and triazolam as hypnotics in the elderly. *Acta Psychiatrica Scandinavica*, 73(329):104–111, 1986.

Beck, A. T., Hollon, S. V., Young, J. E., et al.: Treatment of depression with cognitive therapy and amitriptyline. *Archives of General Psychiatry*, 42:142, 1985.

Benedek, E. T.: Treatment of the female offender: One facility's experience. In W. H. Reid (Ed.), *Treatment of Antisocial Syndromes*. New York: Van Nostrand Reinhold, 1981.

Benson, D. M., Stuss, D. T., Naeser, M. A., et al.: The long-term effects of prefrontal leukotomy. *Archives of Neurology*, 38:165–169, 1981.

Beresin, E., & Gordon, C.: Emergency ward management of the borderline patient. *General Hospital Psychiatry*, 3:237–244, 1981.

Bergman, B., Damber, J. E., Littbrand, B., et al.: Sexual function in prostatic cancer patients treated with radiotherapy, orchiectomy or estrogens. *British Journal of Urology*, 56(1):64–69, 1984.

Berlant, J. L.: Neuroleptics and reserpine in refractory psychoses. *Journal of Clinical Psychopharmacology*, 6(3):180–184, 1986.

Berlin, F. S., & Meinecke, C. F.: Treatment of sex offenders with antiandrogenic medication: Conceptualization, review of treatment modalities, and preliminary findings. *American Journal of Psychiatry*, 138(5):601–607, 1981.

Berman, E., & Wolpert, E. A.: Intractable manic-depressive psychosis with rapid cycling in an eighteen-year-old woman successfully treated with electroconvulsive therapy. *Journal of Nervous and Mental Disease*, 175(4):236–239, 1987.

Biehl, H., Maurer, K., Schubart, C., et al.: Prediction of outcome and utilization of medical services in a prospective study of first onset schizophrenics. Results of a prospective 5-year follow-up study. *European Archives of Psychiatry and Neurological Science*, 236(3):139–147, 1986.

Billiard, M.: The Kleine-Levin syndrome. In W. P. Koella (Ed.), *Sleep*. Basel: S. Karger, 1981, pp. 124–127.

Billiard, M., Guilleminault, C., & Dement, W. C.: A menstruation-linked periodic hypersomnia. *Neurology*, 25:436–443, 1975.

Bixler, E. O., Kales, J. D., Scharf, M. D., et al.: Incidence of sleep disorders in medical practice: A physician survey. In M. H. Chace, M. Mitler, & P. L. Walter (Eds.), *Sleep Research*. Los Angeles: UCLA BIS/BRI 5:160, 1976.

Blackwell, B.: Antidepressant drugs. In M. N. G. Dukes (Ed.), *Meyler's Side Effects of Drugs, Tenth Edition*. Amsterdam: Excerpta Medica, 1984.

Blackwell, B.: Side effects of antidepressant drugs. In R. E. Hales & A. J. Frances (Eds.), *Psychiatry Update, American Psychiatric Association Annual Review, Volume 6*. Washington, D.C.: American Psychiatric Press, 1987, pp. 724–745.

Bliss, E. L.: Multiple personalities. A report of fourteen cases with implications for schizophrenia and hysteria. *Archives of General Psychiatry*, 37(12):1388–1397, 1980.

Blue, F. R.: Use of directive therapy treatment of depersonalization neurosis. *Psychological Reports*, 45: 904–906, 1979.

Bootzin, R. R., & Nicassio, P. N.: Behavior treatments for insomnia. In M. Hersen, R. Eisler, & P. Miller (Eds.), *Progress in Behavior Modification*. New York: Academic Press, 1978.

Bradford, J. M., & Tawlak, A.: Sadistic homosexual pedophilia: Treatment with cyproterone acetate—a single case study. *Canadian Journal of Psychiatry*, 32(1):22–30, 1987.

Branbilla, F., Aguglia, D., Massironi, R., et al.: Neuropeptide therapies in chronic schizophrenia: Trh and vasopressin administration. *Neuropsychobiology* (Switzerland), 15(3–4):114–121, 1986.

Branchy, M. H., Branchy, L. B., & Richardson, M. A.: Effects of neuroleptic adjustment on clinical condition and tardive dyskinesia in schizophrenic patients. *American Journal of Psychiatry*, 138: 608–612, 1981.

Brantley, J. T., & Wise, T. N.: Antiandrogenic treatment of a gender-dysphoric transvestite. *Journal of Sex & Marital Therapy*, 11(2):109–112, 1985.

Braunstein, G. D.: Endocrine causes of impotence. Optimistic outlook for restoration of potency. *Postgraduate Medicine*, 74(4):207–217, 1983.

Bräutigan, W.: Aspects of therapy in psychosomatic medicine. *Psychotherapy and Psychosomatics*, 32:41–51, 1979.

Bridge, T. P., & Wyatt, R. J.: Paraphrenia: Paranoid states of late life. II. American Research. *Journal of the American Geriatric Society*, 28(5):201–205, 1980.

Brizer, D. A., Hartman, N., Sweeney, J., et al.: Effect of methadone plus neuroleptics on treatment-resistant chronic paranoid schizophrenia. *American Journal of Psychiatry*, 142(9):1106–1107, 1985.

Brown, L. S.: Confronting internalized oppression in sex therapy with lesbians. *Journal of Homosexuality*, 12(3–4):99–107, 1986.

Brownell, L. G., West, P., Sweatman, P., et al.: Protriptyline in obstructive sleep apnea. *New England Journal of Medicine*, 307: 1037–1042, 1982.

Bucci, L.: The negative symptoms of schizophrenia and the monoamine oxidase inhibitors. *Psychopharmacology* (Berlin), 91(1):104–108, 1987.

Buigues, J., & Vallejo, J.: Therapeutic response to phenelzine in patients with panic disorder and agoraphobia with panic attacks. *Journal of Clinical Psychiatry*, 48(2):55–59, 1987.

Bumpass, E. R., Brix, R. J., & Preston, B.: A community-based program for juvenile firesetters. *Hospital and Community Psychiatry*, 36(5):529–533, 1985.

Capponi, R., Hormazabal, L., & Schmid-Burgk, W.: Diclofensine and imipramine. A double-blind comparative trial in depressive out-patients. *Neuropsychobiology*, 14(4):173–180, 1985.

Carney, F.: Inpatient treatment programs. In W. H. Reid (Ed.), *The Psychopath: A Comprehensive Study of Antisocial Disorders and Behaviors*. New York: Brunner/Mazel, 1978.

Carpenter, W. T., Jr., & Heinrichs, D. W.: Intermittent psychotherapy of schizophrenia. In J. M. Kane (Ed.), *Drug Maintenance Strategies in Schizophrenia*. Washington, D.C.: American Psychiatric Press, 1984.

Carpenter, W. T., Jr., Heinrichs, D. W., & Hanlon, T. E.: Interpersonal and pharmacologic treatment in schizophrenia: A comparative study of new approaches. *Psychopharmacology Bulletin*, 22(3):854–859, 1986.

Casas, M., Alvarez, E., Duro, T., et al.: Antiandrogenic treatment of obsessive-compulsive neurosis. *Acta Psychiatrica Scandinavica*, 73(2):221–222, 1986.

Casley-Smith, J. R., Casley-Smith, J. R., Johnson, A. F., et al.: Benzo-pyrones and the treatment of chronic schizophrenic diseases. *Psychiatry Research*, 18(3):367–373, 1986.

Chandler, G. M., Burck, H. D., & Sampson, J. P., Jr.: A generic computer program for systematic desensitization: Description, construction, and case study. *Journal of Behavioral Therapy and Experimental Psychiatry*, 17(3):171–174, 1986.

Charney, D. S., & Heninger, G. R.: Noradrenergic function and the mechanism of action of antianxiety treatment. I and II: The effect of long-term alprazolam treatment; the effect of long-term imipramine treatment. *Archives of General Psychiatry*, 42(5):458–467, 473–481, 1985.

Charney, D. S., Woods, S. W., Goodman, W. K., et al.: Drug treatment of panic disorder: The comparative efficacy of imipramine, alprazolam and trazodone. *Journal of Clinical Psychiatry*, 47(12):580–586, 1986.

Chen, H. C., Hsie, M. T., & Shibuya, T. K.: Suanzaorentang vs. diazepam: A controlled double-blind study in anxiety. *International Journal of Clinical Pharmacology, Therapy & Toxicology* (West Germany), 24(12):646–650, 1986.

Chessick, R. D.: Intensive psychotherapy of a borderline patient. *Archives of General Psychiatry*, 39:413–419, 1982.

Chodoff, P.: The therapy of hysterical personality disorders. In J. H. Masserman (Ed.), *Current Psychiatric Therapies, Volume 21*. New York: Grune & Stratton, 1982, pp. 59–65.

Cierpka, M.: Zur psychodynamik der neurotisch bedingten kleptomanie. *Psychiatr Prax.*, 13(3):94–103, 1986.

Clark, B. G., Jue, S. G., Dawson, G. W., et al.: Loprazolam: A preliminary review of its pharmacodynamic and pharmacokinetic properties and therapeutic efficacy in insomnia. *Drugs* 31:500–516, 1986.

Cleckley, H: *The Mask of Sanity (5th ed.)*. St. Louis: C. V. Mosby, 1976.

Climo, L. H.: Treatment-resistant catatonic stupor and combined lithium-neuroleptic therapy: A case report. *Journal of Clinical Psychopharmacology*, 5 (3):166–170, 1985.

Coccaro, E. F., & Siever, L. J.: Second generation antidepressants: A comparative review. *Journal of Clinical Pharmacology*, 25:241–260, 1985.

Cohen, L. J., Shapiro, E., Manson, J. E., et al.: The high cost of treating a psychiatric disorder as a medical/surgical illness. *Psychosomatics*, 26(5):453–455, 1985.

Cohen, S. I.: Updating the model for psychosomatic problems. *Psychotherapy and Psychosomatics*, 32:72–90, 1979.

Cole, J. O., Salomon, M., Gunderson, J., et al.: Drug therapy in borderline patients. *Comprehensive Psychiatry*, 25(3):249–262, 1984.

Cole, M.: Sex therapy—A critical appraisal. *British Journal of Psychiatry*, 147:337–351, 1985.

Coleman, R. M.: Periodic movements in sleep (nocturnal myoclonus) and restless leg syndrome. In C. Guilleminault (Ed.), *Sleeping and Waking Disorder: Indications and Techniques* (pp. 265–296). Menlo Park, CA: Addison-Wesley, 1982.

Coleman, R. M., Roffwarg, H. P., Kennedy, S. J., et al.: Sleep-wake disorders based on a polysomnographic diagnosis: A national cooperative study. *Journal of the American Medical Association,* 247:997–1003, 1982.

Coons, P. M.: Treatment progress in twenty patients with multiple personality disorder. *Journal of Nervous and Mental Disease,* 174(12):715–721, 1986a.

Coons, P. M.: Child abuse and multiple personality disorder: Review of the literature and suggestions for treatment. *Child Abuse and Neglect* (England), 10(4):455–462, 1986b.

Coppen, A., Abou-Saleh, M. T., Nilln, P., et al.: Lithium continuation therapy following electroconvulsive therapy. *British Journal of Psychiatry,* 139:284–287, 1981.

Coppen, A., Chaudhry, S., & Swade, C.: Folic acid enhances lithium prophylaxis. *Journal of Affective Disorders,* 10(1):9–13, 1986.

Cordingley, G. J., Dean, B. C., & Hallett, C.: A multi-centre, double-blind parallel trial of bromazepam (lexotan) and lorazepam to compare the acute benefit-risk ratio in the treatment of patients with anxiety. *Current Medical Research and Opinion,* 9(7):505–510, 1985.

Coryell, W., Lavori, T., Endicott, J., et al.: Outcome in schizoaffective, psychotic, and non-psychotic depression. Course during a six-to-twenty-four-month follow-up. *Archives of General Psychiatry,* 41(8):787–791, 1984.

Cotten-Huston, A. L., & Wheeler, K. A.: Preorgasmic group treatment: Assertiveness marital adjustment and sexual function in women. *Journal of Sex & Marital Therapy,* 9(4):296–302, 1983.

Cottraux, J. A., Bouvard, M., Claustrat, B., et al.: Abnormal dexamethasone suppression test in primary obsessive-compulsive patients: A confirmatory report. *Psychiatry Research,* 13(2):159–165, 1984.

Covi, L., Lipman, R. S., Roth, D., et al.: Cognitive group psychotherapy in depression: A pilot study. *American Journal of Psychiatry,* in press.

Critchley, M.: Periodic hypersomnia and megaphagia in adolescent males. *Brain,* 85:628–656, 1962.

Croughan, J. L., Saghir, M., Cohen, R., et al.: A comparison of treated and untreated male cross-dressers. *Archives of Sexual Behavior,* 10(6):515–528, 1981.

Csanalosi, I., Schweizer, E., Case, W. G., et al.: Gepirone in anxiety: A pilot study. *Journal of Clinical Psychopharmacology,* 7(1):31–33, 1987.

Cytrynbaum, S., & Ken, K.: The Connecticut wilderness program: A preliminary report. State of Connecticut, Council on Human Services, Hartford, Connecticut, 1975.

Daghestani, A. N.: Impotence associated with compulsive gambling. *Journal of Clinical Psychiatry,* 48(3):115–116, 1987.

Dalton, R., Haslett, N., & Baul, G.: Alternative therapy with a recalcitrant firesetter. *Journal of the American Academy of Child Psychiatry,* 25(5):715–717, 1986.

D'Angelo, D. J., & Wolowitz, H. M.: Defensive constellation and styles of recovery from schizophrenic episodes. *Hillside Journal of Clinical Psychiatry,* 8(1):3–14, 1986.

de la Fuente, J. R., Verlanga, C., & Leon-Andrade, C.: Mania induced by tricyclic MAOI combination therapy in bipolar treatment-resistant disorder: Case reports. *Journal of Clinical Psychiatry,* 47(1):40–41, 1986.

De Luca, R. V., & Holborn, S. W.: A comparison of relaxation training and competing response training to eliminate hair-pulling and nailbiting. *Journal of Behavioral Therapy and Experimental Psychiatry,* 15(1):67–70, 1984.

Del Zompo, M., Bocchetta, A., Piccardi, M. P., et al.: Dopamine agonists in the treatment of schizophrenia. *Progress in Brain Research,* 65:41–48, 1986.

den Boer, J. A., Verhoeven, W. M., & Westenberg, H. G.: Remoxipride in schizophrenia. A preliminary report. *Acta Psychiatrica Scandanavica,* 74(4):409–414, 1986.

DePaulo, J. R., Jr., Correa, E. I., & Sapir, D. G.: Renal function and lithium: A longitudinal study. *American Journal of Psychiatry*, 143(7):892–895, 1986.

Dickey, B., Cannon, N. L., McGuire, T. G., et al.: The quarterway house: A two-year cost study of an experimental residential program. *Hospital and Community Psychiatry*, 37(11):1136–1143, 1986.

Dietzel, M., Saletu, B., Lesch, O. M., et al.: Light treatment in depressive illness. Polysomnographic psychometric and neuroendocrinological findings. *European Neurology*, 25(Supplement 2):93–103, 1986.

Doane, J. A., Goldstein, M. J., Miklowitz, D. J., et al.: The impact of individual and family treatment on the affective climate of the families of schizophrenics. *British Journal of Psychiatry*, 148:279–287, 1986.

Dominguez, R. A., Goldstein, B. J., Jacobson, A. F., et al.: Comparative efficacy of estazolam, flurazepam and placebo in outpatients with insomnia. *Journal of Clinical Psychiatry*, 47:362–365, 1986.

Donlon, P. T., Hopkin, J. T., Tupin, J. P., et al.: Haloperidol for acute schizophrenic patients: An evaluation of three oral regimens. *Archives of General Psychiatry*, 37(6):691–695, 1980.

Dossing, M., & Andreasen, B.: Drug-induced liver disease in Denmark: An analysis of 572 cases of hepatotoxicity reported to the Danish Board of Adverse Reactions to Drugs. *Scandinavian Journal of Gastroenterology*, 17:205–211, 1982.

Dowd, E. T., & Swoboda, J. S.: Paradoxical interventions in behavior therapy. *Journal of Behavioral Therapy and Experimental Psychiatry*, 15(3):229–234, 1984.

Drake, R. E., Gates, C., & Cotton, E. G.: Suicide among schizophrenics: A comparison of attemptors and completed suicides. *British Journal of Psychiatry*, 149:784–787, 1986.

Drake, R. E., & Sederer, L. I.: Inpatient psychosocial treatment of chronic schizophrenia: Negative effects and current guidelines. *Hospital and Community Psychiatry*, 37(9):897–901, 1986a.

Drake, R. E., & Sederer, L. I.: The adverse effects of intensive treatment of chronic schizophrenia. *Comprehensive Psychiatry*, 27(4):313–326, 1986b.

Dubovsky, S. L., Franks, R. D., Allen, S., et al.: Calcium antagonists in mania: A double blind study of verapamil. *Psychiatry Research*, 18(4):309–320, 1986.

Dunbar, G. C., Naarala, M., & Hiltumen, H.: A double-blind group comparison of mianserin and clomipramine in the treatment of mildly depressed psychiatric outpatients. *Acta Psychiatrica Scandinavica*, 320 (Supplements):60–66, 1985.

Dunner, D. L., Ishiki, D., Avery, D. H., et al.: Effect of alprazolam and diazepam on anxiety and panic attacks in panic disorder: A controlled study. *Journal of Clinical Psychiatry*, 47(9):458–460, 1986.

Earle, J. R., Jr., & Folks, D. G.: Factitious disorder and coexisting depression: A report of successful psychiatric consultation and case management. *General Hospital Psychiatry*, 8(6):448–450, 1986.

el-Bayoumi, M., el-Sherbini, O., & Mostafa, M.: Impotence in diabetics: Organic vs psychogenic factors. *Urology*, 24(5):459–463, 1984.

Elliott, F. A.: Neurological aspects of antisocial behavior. In W. H. Reid (Ed.), *The Psychopath: A Comprehensive Study of Antisocial Disorders and Behaviors*. New York: Brunner/Mazel, 1978.

Emrich, H. M., Dose, M., & von Zerssen, D.: The use of sodium valproate, carbamazepine, and oxcarbazepine in patients with affective disorders. *Journal of Affective Disorders*, 8(3):243–250, 1985.

Essa, M.: Grief as a crisis: Psychotherapeutic interventions with elderly bereaved. *American Journal of Psychotherapy*, 40(2):243–251, 1986.

Evans, D. L., Davidson, J., & Raft, D.: Early and late side effects of phenelzine. *Journal of Clinical Psychopharmacology*, 2:208–210, 1982.

Evans, D. L., Strawn, S. K., Haggerty, J. J., Jr., et al.: Appearance of mania in drug-resistant bipolar depressed patients after treatment with L-triiodothyromine. *Journal of Clinical Psychiatry*, 47(10):521–522, 1986.

Everaerd, W., & Dekker, J.: Treatment of male sexual dysfunction: Sex therapy compared to the systematic desensitization and rational emotive therapy. *Behaviour Research and Therapy*, 23(1):13–25, 1985.

Falcon, S., Ryan, C., Chamberlain, K., et al.: Tricyclics: Possible treatment for posttraumatic stress disorder. *Journal of Clinical Psychiatry*, 46(9):385–388, 1985.

Faraone, S. V., Brown, W. A., & Laughren, T. P.: Serum neuroleptic levels, prolactin levels, and relapse: A two year study of schizophrenic outpatients. *Journal of Clinical Psychiatry*, 48(4):151–154, 1987.

Faraone, S. V., Curran, J. P., Laughren, T., et al.: Neuroleptic bioavailability, psychosocial factors, and clinical status: A one year study of schizophrenic outpatients after dose reduction. *Psychiatry Research* (Ireland), 19(4):311–322, 1986.

Fenves, A. Z., Emmett, M., & White, M. G.: Lithium intoxications associated with acute renal failure. *Southern Medical Journal*, 77(11):1472–1474, 1984.

Fichten, C. S., Libman, E., & Brender, W.: Methodological issues in the study of sex therapy: Effective components in the treatment of secondary orgasmic dysfunction. *Journal of Sex & Marital Therapy*, 9(3):191–202, 1983.

Finkel, M. J.: Phenytoin revisited. *Clinical Therapeutics*, 6(5):577–591, 1984.

Fogelson, D. L., Marder, S. R., & van Putten, T.: Dialysis for schizophrenia: Review of clinical trials and implications for further research. *American Journal of Psychiatry*, 137(5):605–607, 1980.

Folks, D. G., & Freeman, A. M., III: Munchausen syndrome and other factitious illness. *Psychiatric Clinics of North America*, 8(2):263–278, 1985.

Fontaine, R., & Chouinard, G.: An open clinical trial of fluoxetine in the treatment of obsessive-compulsive disorder. *Journal of Clinical Psychopharmacology*, 6(2):98–101, 1986.

Fontaine, R., Mercier, T., Veaudry, T., et al.: Bromazepam and lorazepam in generalized anxiety: A placebo-controlled study with measurement of blood plasma concentrations. *Acta Psychiatrica Scandinavica*, 74(5):451–458, 1986.

Frances, A., & Carpenter, W. T., Jr.: A schizophrenic patient who resists phenythiazines. *Hospital and Community Psychiatry*, 34(2):115–116, 1983.

Frances, A., & Wise, T. N.: Treating a man who wears women's clothes. *Hospital and Community Psychiatry*, 38(3):233–234, 1987.

Freund, K.: Therapeutic sex drive reduction. *Acta Psychiatrica Scandinavica*, 287(Supplement):5–38, 1980.

Freund, K., & Blanchard, R.: The concept of courtship disorder. *Journal of Sex & Marital Therapy*, 12(2):79–92, 1986.

Freund, K., Scher, H., & Hucker, S.: The courtship disorders: A further investigation. *Archives of Sexual Behavior*, 13(2):133–139, 1984.

Frosch, J. P.: The treatment of antisocial and borderline personality disorders. *Hospital and Community Psychiatry*, 34(3):243–248, 1983.

Gagne, P.: Treatment of sex offenders with medroxyprogesterone acetate. *American Journal of Psychiatry*, 138(5):644–646, 1981.

Galatzer-Levy, R. M.: The opening phase of psychotherapy of hypochondriacal states. *International Journal of Psychoanalytic Psychotherapy*, 9:389–413, 1982.

Ganzarain, R.: Some key issues in the group psychotherapy of narcissistic and borderline patients: Introduction. *International Journal of Group Psychotherapy*, 32(1):3–7, 1982.

Garbutt, J. C., & Loosen, P. T.: A dramatic behavioral response to thyrotropin-releasing hormone following low-dose neuroleptics. *Psychoneuroendocrinology*, 9(3):311–314, 1984.

Gardner, B. L., & Cowdry, R. W.: Positive effects of carbamazepine on behavioral dyscontrol in borderline personality disorder. *American Journal of Psychiatry*, 143(4):519–522, 1986.

Gardos, G., & Casey, B.: *Tardive Dyskinesia and Affective Disorders.* Washington, D.C.: American Psychiatric Press, 1984.

Gelenberg, A. J., & Gibson, C. J.: Tyrosine for the treatment of depression. *Nutrition and Health*, 3(3):163–173, 1984.

Gerner, R. H.: Present status of drug therapy of depression in late life. *Journal of Affective Disorders*, 1(Supplement):S23–S31, 1985.

Getto, C. J.: V Codes for conditions not attributable to a mental disorder that are a focus of treatment. In J. H. Greist, J. W. Jefferson, & R. L. Spitzer (Eds.), *Treatment of Mental Disorders.* New York: Oxford University Press, 1982.

Getto, C. J., & Ochitill, H.: Psychogenic pain disorder. In J. H. Griest, J. W. Jefferson, & R. L. Spitzer (Eds.), *Treatment of Mental Disorders.* New York: Oxford University Press, 1982.

Ghadirian, A. M., & Lalinec-Michaud, M.: Report of a patient with lithium-related alopecia and psoriasis. *Journal of Clinical Psychiatry*, 47(4):212–213, 1986.

Glick, I. D., Fleming, L., DeChillo, N., et al.: A controlled study of transitional daycare for non-chronically-ill patients. *American Journal of Psychiatry*, 143(12):1551–1556, 1986.

Glover, J. H.: A case of kleptomania treated by covert sensitization. *British Journal of Clinical Psychology*, 24(Part 3):213–214, 1985.

Goldberg, H. L., Rickels, K., & Finnerty, R.: Treatment of neurotic depression with a new antidepressant. *Journal of Clinicial Psychopharamacology*, 1(6, Supplement):35S–38S, 1981.

Goldberg, M. A.: The treatment of Kleine-Levine syndrome with lithium. *Canadian Journal of Psychiatry*, 28:491–493, 1983.

Goldberg, S. C., Schulz, S. C., Schulz, P. M., et al.: Borderline and schizotypal personality disorders treated with low-dose thiothixene vs placebo. *Archives of General Psychiatry*, 43(7):680–686, 1986.

Goldman, H. W., Cooper, I. S., Simpson, G. M., et al.: Reversal of severe tardive dyskinesia and dystonia following bilateral CT-guided stereotactic thalatomy (abstract). *Fourth World Congress of Biological Psychiatry.* Philadelphia, Pa., 1985.

Goodnick, P. J., Fieve, R. R., Schlagel, A., et al.: Predictors of interepisode symptoms and relapse in affective disorder patients treated with lithium carbonate. *American Journal of Psychiatry*, 144(3):367–369, 1987.

Goodwin, F. K., Prange, A., Post, R., et al.: Potentiation of antidepressant effects by L-triiodothyronine in tricyclic non-responders. *American Journal of Psychiatry*, 139:34–38, 1982.

Graber, B. G.: Demystifying "sex therapy." *American Journal of Psychotherapy*, 35(4):481–488, 1981.

Graber, B. G.: *Circumvaginal musculature and sexual function.* Basel, Switzerland: S. Karger, 1982.

Gralnick, A.: The future of the chronic schizophrenic patient: Prediction and recommendations. *American Journal of Psychotherapy*, 40(3):419–429, 1986.

Granier, F., Girard, M., Schmitt, L., et al.: Depression and anxiety: Mianserin and nomifensime compared in a double-blind multicentre trial. *Acta Psychiatrica Scandinavica*, 320(Supplement):67–74, 1985.

Greben, S. E.: The multi-dimensional inpatient treatment of severe character disorders. *Canadian Journal of Psychiatry*, 28(2):97–101, 1983.

Greenblatt, D. J., Harmatz, G. S., Zinny, M. A., et al.: Effect of gradual withdrawal on the rebound sleep disorder after discontinuation of triazolam. *New England Journal of Medicine*, 317:722–728, 1987.

Greil, W., Stoltzenburg, M. C., Mairhofer, M. L., et al.: Lithium dosage in the elderly. A study with matched age groups. *Journal of Affective Disorders*, 9(1):1–4, 1985.

Grigsby, J. T.: Use of imagery in the treatment of posttraumatic stress disorder. *Journal of Nervous and Mental Disease*, 175(1):55–59, 1987.

Gross, G., & Huber, G.: Classification and prognosis schizophrenic disorders in light of the Bonn follow-up studies. *Psychopathology*, 19(1–2):50–59, 1986.

Guilleminault, C., Carskadon, M., & Dement, W. C.: On the treatment of rapid eye movement narcolepsy. *Archives of Neurology*, 30:90–93, 1974.

Guilleminault, C., & Flagg, W.: Effects of baclofen on sleep-related periodic leg movements. *Annals of Neurology*, 15:234–239, 1984.

Guilleminault, C., Nino-Murcia, G., Heldt, G., et al.: Alternative treatment to tracheostomy in obstructive sleep apnea syndrome: Nasal continuous positive airway pressure in young children. *Pediatrics*, 78:797–802, 1986.

Guilleminault, C., Quera-Salva, M. A., Nino-Murcia, G., et al.: Central sleep apnea and partial obstruction of the airway. *Annals of Neurology*, 21:465–469, 1987.

Haggerty, J., Jr., & Jackson, R.: Mania following change from trazodone to imipramine. *Journal of Clinical Psychopharmacology*, 5(6):342–343, 1985.

Handwerker, J. V., Jr., & Palmer, R. F.: Clonidine and the treatment of "restless leg" syndrome. *New England Journal of Medicine*, 313:1228–1229, 1985.

Harrison, W. M., Rabkin, J. G., Ehrhardt, A. A., et al.: Effects of antidepressant medication on sexual functions: A controlled study. *Journal of Clinical Psychopharmacology*, 6(3):144–149, 1986.

Hartman, L. M.: Effects of sex and marital therapy on sexual interaction and marital happiness. *Journal of Sex & Marital Therapy*, 9(2):137–151, 1983a.

Hartman, L. M.: Resistance in directive sex therapy: Recognition and management. *Journal of Sex & Marital Therapy*, 9(4):283–295, 1983b.

Hauri, P. J.: *The Sleep Disorders*. Kalamazoo, MI: Upjohn, 1977, pp. 1–76.

Hauri, P. J.: *The Sleep Disorders: Current Concepts*. Kalamazoo, MI: Upjohn Scope Publications, 1982, p. 54.

Hauri, P. J.: Primary sleep disorders and insomnia. In T. L. Riley (Ed.), *Clinical Aspects of Sleep Disturbance*. London: Butterworths 5:98–100, 1985.

Hawton, K., & Catalan, J.: Prognostic factors in sex therapy. *Behaviour Research and Therapy Journal*, 24(4):377–385, 1986.

Heiman, J. R., & LoPiccolo, J.: Clinical outcome of sex therapy. Effects of daily vs weekly treatment. *Archives of General Psychiatry*, 40(4):443–449, 1983.

Hening, W. A., Walters, A., Kavey, N., et al.: Dyskinesias while awake and periodic movements in sleep in restless syndrome: Treatment with opioids. *Neurology*, 36:1363–1366, 1986.

Herrmann, W. M., & Beach, R. C.: Pharmacotherapy for sexual offenders: Review of the actions of antiandrogens with special references to their psychic effects. *Modern Problems in Pharmacopsychiatry*, 15:182–194, 1980.

Hirschfeld, R. M., Klerman, G. L., Keller, M. B., et al.: Personality of recovered patients with bipolar affective disorder. *Journal of Affective Disorders*, 11(1):81–89, 1986.

Hogarty, G. E., Anderson, C. M., Reiss, D. J., et al.: Family psychoeducation, social skills training and maintenance chemotherapy in the aftercare treatment of schizophrenia. I. One-year effects of a controlled study on relapse and expressed emotion. *Archives of General Psychiatry*, 43(7):633–642, 1986.

Holcomb, W. R.: Stress inoculation therapy with anxiety and stress disorders of acute psychiatric patients. *Journal of Clinical Psychology*, 42(6):864–872, 1986.

Hollister, L. E.: Pharmacotherapeutic considerations in anxiety disorders. *Journal of Clinical Psychiatry*, 47(June Supplement):33–36, 1986.

Holman, S. L.: A group program for borderline mothers and their toddlers. *International Journal of Group Psychotherapy*, 35(1):79–93, 1985.

Hoon, P. W.: Physiologic assessment of sexual response in women: The unfulfilled promise. *Clinical Obstetrics and Gynecology,* 27(3):767–780, 1984.

Horne, D. J., McCormack, H. M., Collins, J. P., et al.: Psychological treatment of phobic anxiety associated with adjuvant chemotherapy. *Medical Journal of Australia,* 145(7):346–348, 1986.

Horowitz, M. J.: Stress-response syndromes: A review of posttraumatic and adjustment disorders. *Hospital and Community Psychiatry,* 37(3):241–249, 1986.

Horowitz, M. J., Marmar, C., Weiss, D. S., et al.: Brief psychotherapy of bereavement reactions. The relationship of process to outcome. *Archives of General Psychiatry,* 41(5):438–448, 1984.

Horwitz, L.: Divergent views on the treatment of borderline patients. *Bulletin of the Menninger Clinic,* 49(6):525–545, 1985.

Hyler, S. B., & Sussman, N.: Chronic factitious disorder with physical symptoms (The Munchausen Syndrome). *Psychiatric Clinics of North America,* 4(2):365–377, 1981.

Hymowitz, P., Frances, A., Jacobsberg, L. B., et al.: Neuroleptic treatment of schizotypal personality disorder. *Comprehensive Psychiatry,* 27(4):267–271, 1986.

Inoue, K., Nakajima, T., & Kato, N.: A longitudinal study of schizophrenia in adolescents. In the one-to-three-year outcome. *Japanese Journal of Psychiatry and Neurology,* 40(2):143–151, 1986.

Insel, T. R., Mueller, E. A. III, Gillin, J. C., et al.: Biological markers in obsessive-compulsive and affective disorders. *Journal of Psychiatric Research,* 18(4):407–423, 1984.

Insel, T. R., Mueller, E. A., Gillin, J. C., et al.: Tricyclic response in obsessive-compulsive disorder. *Progress in Neuropsychopharmacological and Biological Psychiatry,* 9(1):25031, 1985.

Insel, T. R., Murphy, D. L., Cohen, R. M., et al.: Obsessive-compulsive disorder. *Archives of General Psychiatry,* 40:605–612, 1983.

International Drug Therapy Newsletter. New hope for tricyclic refractory unipolar depressives? 16(7):25–27, 1981.

International Drug Therapy Newsletter: Buspirone: A new generation anxiolytic. 19:1–4, 1984.

Jaeger, A., Sauder, P., Kopfreschmitt, J., et al.: Toxicokinetics of lithium intoxication treated by hemodialysis. *Journal of Toxicology and Clinical Toxicology,* 23(7–8):501–517, 1985.

Jann, M. W., Saklad, S. R., Ereshefsky, L., et al.: Effects of smoking on haloperidol and reduced haloperidol plasma concentrations and haloperidol clearance. *Psychopharmacology* (Berlin), 19(4):468–470, 1986.

Jansson, L., Jerremalm, A., & Ost, L. G.: Follow-up of agoraphobic patients treated with exposure in vivo or applied relaxation. *British Journal of Psychiatry,* 149: 486–490, 1986.

Jarrett, R. B., & Rush, A. J.: Psychotherapeutic approaches for depression. In N. R. Michaels, J. O. Cavenar, Jr., et al. (Eds.), *Psychiatry, Volume 1.* Philadelphia: J. B. Lippincott, 1986.

Jefferson, J. W., Greist, J. H., & Ackerman, D. L.: *Lithium Encyclopedia for Clinical Practice.* Washington, D.C.: American Psychiatric Press, 1983.

Jelinek, J. M., & Williams, T.: Post-traumatic stress disorder and substance abuse in Vietnam combat veterans: Treatment problems, strategies and recommendations. *Journal of Substance Abuse Treatment,* 1(2):87–97, 1984.

Jenkins, S. C., & Maruta, T.: Therapeutic use of propranolol for Intermittent Explosive Disorder. *Mayo Clinic Proceedings,* 62(3):204–214, 1987.

Jensen, S. B.: Sexual dysfunction in younger insulin-treated diabetic females: A comparative study. *Diabete et Metabolisme,* 11(5):278–282, 1985.

Joffe, R. T., & Brown, P.: Clinical and biological correlates of sleep deprivation in depression. *Canadian Journal of Psychiatry,* 29(6):530–536, 1984.

Johansen, K. H.: The impact of patients with chronic character pathology on a hospital inpatient unit. *Hospital and Community Psychiatry,* 34(9):842–846, 1983.

Johnson, B., Geller, J., Gordon, J., et al.: Group psychotherapy with schizophrenic patients: Pairing group. *International Journal of Group Psychotherapy*, 36(1):75–96, 1986.

Johnson, C., Shenoy, R. S., & Langer, S.: Relaxation therapy for somatoform disorders. *Hospital and Community Psychiatry*, 32(6):423–424, 1981.

Johnson, S. B., Alvarez, W. A., & Freinhar, J. P.: A case of massive rhabdomyolysis following molindone administration. *Journal of Clinical Psychiatry*, 47(12):607–608, 1986.

Joint Commission on Accreditation of Hospitals: *Accreditation Manual for Hospitals*. Chicago, 1988.

Jorgensen, P.: Long-term course of acute reactive paranoid psychosis. A follow-up study. *Acta Psychiatrica Scandanavica*, 71(1):30–37, 1985.

Jorgensen, P., & Munk-Jorgensen, P.: Paranoid psychosis in the elderly. A follow-up study. *Acta Psychiatrica Scandinavica*, 72(4):358–363, 1985.

Kales, A., & Kales, J. D.: *Evaluation and Treatment of Insomnia*. New York: Oxford University Press, 1984.

Kales, A., Soldatos, C. R., Bixler, E. O., et al.: Narcolepsy-cataplexy. II. Psychosocial consequences and associated psychopathology. *Archives of Neurology*, 39:169–171, 1982.

Kales, A., Soldatos, C. R., Cadieux, R., et al.: Propranolol in the treatment of narcolepsy. *Annals of Internal Medicine*, 91:742–743, 1979.

Kane, J. M., & Smith, J. M.: Tardive dyskinesia: Prevalence and risk factors. *Archives of General Psychiatry*, 39:473–481, 1982.

Kane, J. M., Woerner, M., Weinhold, P., et al.: Incidence of tardive dyskinesia: Five year data from the prospective study. *Psychopharmacology Bulletin*, 20:387–389, 1984.

Kaplan, C. A.: The challenge of working with patients diagnosed as having a borderline personality disorder. *Nursing Clinics of North America*, 21(3):429–438, 1986.

Kaplan, H. S.: *The New Sex Therapy*. New York: Brunner/Mazel, 1974.

Kaplan, H. S.: *Disorders of Sexual Desire*. New York: Brunner/Mazel, 1979.

Kaplan, H. S.: Psychosexual dysfunctions. In R. M. Michaels & J. O. Cavenar (Eds.), *Psychiatry, Volume 1*. Philadelphia: J. B. Lippincott, 1986.

Karacan, I., Moore, C. A., & Williams, R. L.: The narcoleptic syndrome. *Psychiatric Annals*, 9(7):377–381, 1979.

Karacan, I., Thornby, J., Anch, M., et al.: Prevalence of sleep disturbance in a primarily urban Florida county. *Social Science and Medicine*, 10:239–244, 1976.

Karasu, T. D.: Psychotherapy of the psychosomatic patient. *American Journal of Psychotherapy*, 33(3):354–364, 1979.

Kartman, L. L.: Music hath charms. . . . *Journal of Gerontological Nursing*, 10(6):20–24, 1984.

Katz, R. J.: Effects of zometapine, a structurally novel antidepressant, in an animal model of depression. *Pharmacology and Biochemical Behavior*, 21(4):487–490, 1984.

Kaufman, K. R., & Okeya, V. L.: Lithium in pregnancy—Avoidance of toxicity. A case report. *Biological Research in Pregnancy and Perinatology*, 6(2):55–58, 1985.

Kazi, H. A.: An open clinical trial with the long-acting neuroleptic zuclopenthixol decanoate in the maintenance treatment of schizophrenia. *Pharmatherapeutica*, 4(9):555–560, 1986.

Keller, M. V., Lavori, P. W., Coryell, W., et al.: Differential outcome of pure manic, mixed/cycling and pure depressive episodes in patients with bipolar illness. *Journal of the American Medical Association*, 255(22):3138–3142, 1986.

Kellner, R.: Psychotherapy in psychosomatic disorders: A survey of controlled studies. *Archives of General Psychiatry*, 32:1021–1030, 1975.

Kellner, R.: Psychotherapeutic strategies in hypochondriasis: A clinical study. *American Journal of Psychotherapy*, 36(2):146–157, 1982a.

Kellner, R.: Disorders of impulse control. In J. H. Greist, J. W. Jefferson, & R. L. Spitzer (Eds.), *Treatment of Mental Disorders*. New York: Oxford University Press, 1982b.

Kellner, R.: Prognosis of treated hypochrondriasis. A clinical study. *Acta Psychiatrica Scandinavica*, 67(2):69–79, 1983.

Kellner, R.: Functional somatic symptoms and hypochondriasis. A survey of empirical studies. *Archives of General Psychiatry*, 42(8):821–833, 1985.

Kentsmith, D. K., & Eaton, M. T.: *Treating Sexual Problems in Medical Practice*. New York: Arco, 1979.

Kernberg, O. F.: Narcissistic personality disorder. In R. M. Michaels & J. O. Cavenar (Eds.), *Psychiatry, Volume I*. Philadelphia: J. B. Lippincott, 1986a.

Kernberg, O. F.: Hysterical and histrionic personality disorders. In R. Michaels & J. O. Cavenar, Jr. (Eds.), *Psychiatry, Volume 1*. Philadelphia: J. B. Lippincott, 1986b.

Khan, A., Jaffe, J. H., Nelson, W. H., et al.: Resolution of neuroleptic malignant syndrome with dantrolene sodium: Case report. *Journal of Clinical Psychiatry*, 46(6):244–246, 1985.

Khuri, R., & Gehi, M.: Psychogenic amenorrhea: An integrated review. *Psychosomatics*, 22(10):883–893, 1981.

Kiev, A.: Cluster analysis profiles of suicide attempts. *American Journal of Psychiatry*, 133(2):150–153, 1976.

Kilmann, P. R., Boland, J. C., Norton, S. P., et al.: Perspectives of sex therapy outcome: A survey of AASECT providers. *Journal of Sex & Marital Therapy*, 12(2):116–138, 1986.

Kimball, C. T.: *The Biopsychosocial Approach to the Patient*. Baltimore: Williams & Wilkins, 1981.

Kimball, R. O.: Wilderness experience program: Final evaluation report. Santa Fe, New Mexico, Health and Environment Department, 1979.

Kinney, J. L.: Nomifensine malleate: A new second-generation antidepressant. *Clinical Pharmacology*, 4(6):625–636, 1984.

Kitchner, I., & Greenstein, R.: Low dose lithium carbonate in the treatment of post-traumatic stress disorder: Brief communication. *Military Medicine*, 150(7):378–381, 1985.

Klar, H.: The setting for psychiatric treatment. In R. E. Hales & A. J. Frances (Eds.), *Psychiatry Update, Annual Review, Volume 6*. Washington, D.C.: American Psychiatric Press, 1987, pp. 336–352.

Klonoff, E. A., Youngner, S. J., Moore, E. J., et al.: Chronic factitious illness: A behavioral approach. *International Journal of Psychiatry and Medicine*, 13(3):173–183, 1983.

Kluft, R. P.: An update on multiple personality disorder. *Hospital and Community Psychiatry*, 38(4):363–373, 1987.

Knobler, H. Y., Itzchaky, S., Emanuel, D., et al.: Trazodone-induced mania. *British Journal of Psychiatry*, 149: 787–789, 1986.

Koehler, K., & Sauer, H.: First rank symptoms as predictors of ECT response in schizophrenia. *British Journal of Psychiatry*, 142:280, 1983.

Koenigsberg, H. W.: Indications for hospitalization in the treatment of borderline patients. *Psychiatric Quarterly*, 56(4):247–258, 1984.

Koles, M. R., & Jenson, W. R.: Comprehensive treatment of chronic firesetting in a severely disordered boy. *Journal of Behavioral Therapy and Experimental Psychiatry*, 16(1):81–85, 1985.

Kolko, D. J.: Multicomponent parental treatment of firesetting in a six-year-old boy. *Journal of Behavioral Therapy and Experimental Psychiatry*, 14(4):349–353, 1983.

Kravitz, H. M., Sabelli, H. C., & Fawcett, J.: Dietary supplements of phenylalanine and other amino acid precursors of brain neuroamines in the treatment of depressive disorders. *Journal of the American Osteopathic Association*, 84(Supplement):119–123, 1984.

Kretsch, R., Goren, Y., & Wasserman, A.: Change patterns of borderline patients in individual and group therapy. *International Journal of Group Therapy*, 37(1):95–112, 1987.

Krishnan, R. R., Davidson, J., & Miller, R.: MAO inhibitor therapy in trichotillomania associated with depression: Case report. *Journal of Clinical Psychiatry,* 45(6):267–268, 1984.

Kuch, K., Swinson, R. P., & Kirby, M.: Post-traumatic stress disorder after car accident. *Canadian Journal of Psychiatry,* 30(6):426–427, 1985.

Lamontagne, Y., & Lesage, A.: Private exposure and covert sensitization in the treatment of exhibitionists. *Journal of Behavioral Therapy and Experimental Psychiatry,* 17(3): 197–201, 1986.

Lanza, U.: The contribution of acupuncture to clinical psychotherapy by means of biofeedback (EMG-BME) training. *Acupuncture & Electrotherapeutics Research,* 11(1):53–57, 1986.

Laws, D. R.: Sexual fantasy alteration: Procedural considerations. *Journal of Behavioral Therapy and Experimental Psychiatry,* 16(1):39–44, 1985.

Lawy, A. J., Sack, R. L., Fredrickson, R. H., et al.: The use of bright light in the treatment of chronobiologic sleep and mood disorders: The phase-response curve. *Psychopharmacology Bulletin,* 19(3):523–525, 1983.

Lawy, A. J., Sack, R. L., & Singer, C. M.: Treating phase-typed chronobiologic sleep and mood disorders using appropriately timed bright artificial light. *Psychopharmacology Bulletin,* 21:368–372, 1985.

Lazara, A.: Conversion symptoms. *New England Journal of Medicine,* 305(13):745–748, 1981.

Lazarus, J. H., McGregor, A. M., Ludgate, M., et al.: Effect of lithium carbonate therapy on thyroid immune status in manic depressive patients: A prospective study. *Journal of Affective Disorders* (Netherlands), 11(2):155–169, 1986.

Lazarus, L. W., Davis, J. M., & Dysken, M. W.: Geriatric depression: A guide to successful therapy. *Geriatrics,* 40(6):43–48, 52–53, 1985.

Ledermann, R.: Narcissistic disorder and its treatment. *Journal of Analytical Psychology,* 27:303–321, 1982.

Lehman, C. R., Ereshefsky, L., Saklad, S. R., & Mings, T. E.: Very high dose loxapine in refractory schizophrenic patients. *American Journal of Psychiatry,* 138:1212–1214, 1981.

Lelliott, P. T., & Monteiro, W. O.: Drug treatment of obsessive-compulsive disorder. *Drugs,* 31(1):75–80, 1986.

Lenox, R. H., Modell, J. G., & Weiner, S.: Acute treatment of manic agitation with lorazepam. *Psychosomatics,* 21(1, Supplement):28–32, 1986.

Lerer, B.: Alternative therapies for biopolar disorder. *Journal of Clinical Psychiatry,* 46(8):309–316, 1985.

Lerer, B., Moore, N., Meyendorff, E., et al.: Carbamazepine vs. lithium in mania: A double-blind study. *Journal of Clinical Psychiatry,* 48(3):89–93, 1987.

Lesser, M. S., Cahan, M., Brenner, R., & Nayak, D.: Dantrolene sodium as a possible prophylactic agent against NMS. *Hillside Journal of Clinical Psychiatry,* 8(1):34–37, 1986.

Levinson, D., & Simpson, G.: EPS with fever: Heterogeneity of the neuroleptic malignant syndrome. *Archives of General Psychiatry,* 43:839–848, 1986.

Levinson, D., & Simpson, G.: Antipsychotic drug side effects. In R. E. Hales & A. J. Frances (Eds.), *Psychiatry Update, Annual Review, Volume 6.* Washington, D.C.: American Psychiatric Press, 1987, pp. 704–723.

Lewis, D. A., & Nasrallah, H. A.: Mania associated with electroconvulsive therapy. *Journal of Clinical Psychiatry,* 47(7):366–367, 1986.

Lewis, J. L., & Winokur, G.: The induction of mania, a natural history study with controls. *Archives of General Psychiatry,* 39: 303–306, 1982.

Lewy, A. J., Sack, R. L., Miller, L. S., et al.: Antidepressants and circadian phase-shifting effects of light. *Science,* 235(4786):352–354, 1987.

Lewy, A. J., Sack, R. L., & Singer, C. M.: Melatonin, light and chronobiological disorders. *Ciba Foundation Symposia,* 117:231–252, 1985.

Libman, E., Fichten, C. S., Brinder, W., et al.: A comparison of three therapeutic formats in the treatment of secondary orgasmic dysfunction. *Journal of Sex & Marital Therapy,* 10(3):147–159, 1984.

Lichstein, T. R.: Caring for the patient with multiple somatic complaints. *Southern Medical Journal,* 79(3):310–314, 1986.

Liebowitz, M. R.: Imipramine in the treatment of panic disorder and its complications. *Psychiatric Clinics of North America,* 8(1):37–47, 1985.

Lindberg, F. H., & Distad, L. J.: Post-traumatic stress disorders in women who experienced childhood incest. *Child Abuse and Neglect,* 9(3):329–334, 1985.

Lindsay, W. R., Gansu, C. V., McLaughlin, E., et al.: A controlled trial of treatments for generalized anxiety. *British Journal of Clinical Psychology,* 26(part 1):3–15, 1987.

Lion, J. R.: Countertransference and other psychotherapy issues. In W. H. Reid (Ed.), *The Treatment of Antisocial Syndromes.* New York: Van Nostrand Reinhold, 1981.

Lisansky, J., Fava, G. A., Buckman, M. T., et al.: Prolactin, amitriptyline, and recovery from depression. *Psychopharmacology* (Berlin), 84(3):331–335, 1984.

LoPiccolo, J., Heiman, J. R., Hogan, D. R., et al.: Effectiveness of single therapist vs. cotherapy teams in sex therapy. *Journal of Consulting and Clinical Psychology,* 53(3):287–294, 1985.

Louie, A. K., & Meltzer, H. Y.: Lithium potentiation of antidepressant treatment. *Journal of Clinical Psychopharmacology,* 4(6):316–321, 1984.

Lowe, M. R., & Batchelor, D. H.: Depot neuroleptics and manic-depressive psychosis. *International Clinical Psychopharmacology* (England), 1(Supplement 1):53–62, 1986.

Lukoff, D., Wallace, C. J., Liberman, R. P., et al.: A holistic program for chronic schizophrenic patients. *Schizophrenia Bulletin,* 12(2):274–282, 1986.

Lybiard, R. B.: Obsessive-compulsive disorder successfully treated with trazodone. *Psychosomatics,* 27(12):858–859, 1986.

Macaskill, N. D.: Therapeutic factors in group therapy with borderline patients. *International Journal of Group Psychotherapy,* 32(1):61–73, 1982.

MacHovec, F. J.: Hypnosis to facilitate recall in psychogen amnesia and fugue states: Treatment variables. *American Journal of Clinical Hypnosis,* 24(1):7–13, 1981.

Mahapatra, R. K., Paul, S. K., Mahapatra, D., et al.: Cardiovascular effects of polycyclic antidepressants. *Angiology,* 37(10):709–717, 1986.

Mahgoub, O. M.: A remarkable response of chronic severe obsessive-compulsive neurosis to phenelzine. *Acta Psychiatrica Scandinavica,* 75(2):222–223, 1987.

Maj, M., Starace, F., Nolfe, G., et al.: Minimum plasma lithium levels required for effective prophylaxis in DSM–III bipolar disorder: A prospective study. *Pharmacopsychiatry* (West Germany), 19(6):420–423, 1986.

Majid, I.: A double-blind comparison of one-daily flupenthixol and mianserin in depressed hospital outpatients. *Pharmatherapeutica,* 4(7):405–410, 1986.

Maletzky, V. M.: *Multiple-monitored Electroconvulsive Therapy.* Boca Raton, FL: CRC, 1981.

Malinow, K. L.: Dependent personality. In J. R. Lion (Ed.), *Personality Disorders: Diagnosis and Management* (Second Edition). Baltimore: Williams & Wilkins, 1981.

Mamelak, M., & Webster, P.: Treatment of narcolepsy and sleep apnea with gamma-hydroxybutyrate: A clinical and polysomnographic case study. *Sleep,* 4:105–111, 1981.

Manchanda, R., & Hirsch, S. R.: Does propranolol have an antipsychotic effect? A placebo-controlled study in acute schizophrenia. *British Journal of Psychiatry,* 148: 701–707, 1986.

Mander, A. J.: Clinical prediction of the outcome of lithium response in bipolar affective disorder. *Journal of Affective Disorders,* 11(1):35–41, 1986.

Marder, S. R., van Putten, T., Mintz, J., et al.: Maintenance therapy in schizophrenia: New findings. In J. M. Kane (Ed.), *Drug Maintenance Strategies in Schizophrenia.* Washington, D.C.: American Psychiatric Press, 1984.

Marks, I. M.: Review of behavioral psychotherapy. I. Obsessive-compulsive disorders. *American Journal of Psychiatry,* 138(5):584–592, 1981a.

Marks, I. M.: Review of behavioral psychotherapy. II: Sexual disorders. *American Journal of Psychiatry*, 138(6):750–756, 1981b.

Marks, I. M.: Behavioral psychotherapy for anxiety disorders. *Psychiatric Clinics of North America*, 8(1):25–35, 1985.

Marmor, J.: The psychodynamic approach in the treatment of sexual problems. In M. R. Zales (Ed.), *Eating, Sleeping, and Sexuality: Treatment of Disorders in Basic Life Functions.* New York: Brunner/Mazel, 1982.

Martin, B. A.: Electroconvulsive therapy: Contemporary standards of practice. *Canadian Journal of Psychiatry*, 31:759–771, 1986.

Martin, W. R., Sloan, J. W., Sapira, J. D., et al.: Physiologic, subjective and behavioral effects of amphetamine, methamphetamine, ephedrine, phenmetrazine and methylphenidate in man. *Clinical Pharmacology & Therapeutics*, 12:245–258, 1971.

Masters, W., & Johnson, V.: *Human Sexual Inadequacy*. Boston: Little, Brown, 1970.

Mattes, J. A.: Metoprolol for intermittent explosive disorder. *American Journal of Psychiatry*, 142(9):1108–1109, 1985.

Mavissakalian, M. M., & Michelson, L.: Agoraphobia: Behavioral and pharmacological treatments. *Psychopharmacology Bulletin*, 18: 91–103, 1982.

Mavissakalian, M., & Michelson, L.: Agoraphobia: Relative and combined effectiveness of therapist-assisted in vivo exposure and imipramine. *Journal of Clinical Psychiatry*, 47(3):117–122, 1986a.

Mavissakalian, M., & Michelson, L.: Two-year follow-up of exposure and imipramine treatment of agoraphobia. *American Journal of Psychiatry*, 143(9):1106–1112, 1986b.

Mawson, B., Marks, I., Ramm, E., et al.: Guided mourning for morbid grief: A controlled study. *British Journal of Psychiatry*, 138: 185–193, 1981.

May, P. R. A., van Putten, T., Jenden, D. J., et al.: Chlorpromazine levels and the outcome of treatment in schizophrenic patients. *Archives of General Psychiatry*, 38: 202–207, 1981.

McCabe, B., & Tsuang, M. T.: Dietary considerations in MAO inhibitor regimens. *Journal of Clinical Psychiatry*, 43:178–181, 1982.

McCann, I. L., & Holmes, D. S.: Influence of aerobic exercise on depression. *Journal of Personality and Social Psychology*, 46(5):1142–1147, 1984.

McConaghy, N., Armstrong, M. S., Blaszczynski, A., et al.: Controlled comparison of aversive therapy and imaginal desensitization in compulsive gambling. *British Journal of Psychiatry*, 142:366–372, 1983.

McCormick, R. A., Russo, A. M., Ramirez, L. F., et al.: Affective disorders among pathological gamblers seeking treatment. *American Journal of Psychiatry*, 141(2):215–218, 1984.

McCreadie, R., Mackie, M., Morrison, D., et al.: Once weekly pimozide vs. fluphenazine decanoate and maintenance therapy in chronic schizophrenia. *British Journal of Psychiatry*, 140:280–286, 1982.

McEvoy, J. P., & Lohr, J. B.: Diazepam for catatonia. *American Journal of Psychiatry*, 141(2):284–285, 1984.

McEvoy, R. D., & Thornton, A. T.: Treatment of obstructive sleep apnea syndrome with nasal continuous positive airway pressure. *Sleep*, 7(4):313–325, 1984.

McGlashan, T. H.: Intensive individual psychotherapy of schizophrenia. A review of techniques. *Archives of General Psychiatry*, 40(8):909–920, 1983.

McGlashan, T. H.: Schizotypal personality disorder. Chestnut Lodge follow-up study: VI. Long-term follow-up perspectives. *Archives of General Psychiatry*, 43(4):329–334, 1986.

McMillan, D. E., Fody, E. P., Couch, L., et al.: Drug holidays and serum haloperidol levels in schizophrenic patients. *General Clinical Psychiatry*, 47(7):373–374, 1986.

McNair, D. M., Kahn, R. J., Frankenthaler, L. M., et al.: Amoxapine and amitriptyline. I. Relative speed of antidepressant action. *Psychopharmacology* (Berlin), 83(2):129–133, 1984a.

McNair, D. M., Kahn, R. J., Frankenthaler, L. M., et al.: Amoxapine and amitriptyline. II. Specificity of cognitive effects during brief treatment of depression. *Psychopharmacology* (Berlin), 83(2):134–139, 1984b.

Meadow, R.: Fictitious epilepsy. *Lancet*, 2(8393):25–28, 1984.

Mellion, M. B.: Exercise therapy for anxiety and depression. 1. Does the evidence justify its recommendation? *Postgraduate Medicine*, 77(3):59–66, 1985.

Meltzer, H. Y., Sommers, A. A., & Luchins, D. J.: The effect of neuroleptics and other psychotropic drugs on negative symptoms in schizophrenia. *Journal of Clinical Psychopharmacology*, 6(6):329–338, 1986.

Mendlewicz, J., Hubain, T. P., & Koumakis, C.: Further investigation of the dexamethasone suppression test in affective illnesses: Relationship to clinical diagnosis and therapeutic response. *Neuropsychobiology*, 12(1):23–26, 1984.

Michelson, L., & Ascher, L. M.: Paradoxical intention in the treatment of agoraphobia and other anxiety disorders. *Journal of Behavioral Therapy and Experimental Psychiatry*, 15(3):215–220, 1984.

Micheroli, R., & Battegay, R.: Ambulatante behandlung von sexualdelinquenten mit cyproteronacetat (Androcur) eime katannestiche untersuchung. *Schweiz Arch. Neurol. Psychiatr.*, 136(5):37–58, 1985.

Mitchell, J. D., & Poplin, M. K.: Antidepressant drug therapy and sexual dysfunction in men: A review. *General Clinical Psychopharmacology*, 3:76–79, 1983.

Mitler, M. M., Browman, C. P., Menn, S. J., et al.: Nocturnal myoclonus: Treatment efficacy of clonazepam and temazepam. *Sleep*, 9(3):385–392, 1986.

Modell, J. G., Lenox, R. H., & Weiner, S.: Inpatient clinical trials of lorazepam for the management of manic agitation. *Journal of Clinical Psychopharmacology*, 5:109–113, 1985.

Moldofsky, H., & Lue, F. A.: The relationship of alpha and delta EEG frequencies to pain and mode in fibrositis patients treated with chlorpromazine and L-tryptophan. *Electroencephalography & Clinical Neurophysiology*, 50:71–80, 1980.

Moldofsky, H., Musisi, S., & Phillipson, E. A.: Treatment of a case of advanced sleep-phase syndrome by phase advance chronotherapy. *Sleep* 9(1):61–65, 1986.

Monroe, R. R.: The problem of impulsivity in personality disturbances. In J. R. Lion (Ed.), *Personality Disorders: Diagnosis and Management* (Second Edition). Baltimore: Williams & Wilkins, 1981.

Montplaisir, J., Godbout, R., Boghen, D., et al.: Familial restless legs with periodic movements in sleep: Electrophysiologic biochemical and pharmacological study. *Neurology*, 35:130–134, 1985.

Mosher, L. R., & Keith, S. J.: Research on the psychosocial treatment of schizophrenia: A summary report. *American Journal of Psychiatry*, 137(5):623–631, 1979.

Moss, E., & Garb, R.: Integrated psychotherapeutic treatment of somatoform and other psychophysiological disorders. *Psychotherapy and Psychosomatics*, 25(2):105–112, 1986.

Mukherjee, S., Rosen, A. M., Caracci, G., et al.: Persistent tardive dyskinesia in bipolar patients. *Archives of General Psychiatry*, 43(4):342–346, 1986.

Muller, Y. L.: Depersonalisation—Symptoms, meaning, therapy. *Acta Psychiatrica Scandinavica*, 66(6):451–458, 1982.

Murphy, E.: General management of depression in late life. *Journal of Affective Disorders*, (Supplement 1):S7–S10, 1985.

Murphy, G. E., Simons, A. D., Wetzle, R. D., et al.: Cognitive therapy and pharmacotherapy: Singly and together in the treatment of depression. *Archives of General Psychiatry*, 41:33, 1984.

Murphy, M. F., & Davis, K. L.: Biological perspectives in chronic pain, depression, and organic mental disorders. *Psychiatric Clinics of North America*, 4(2):223–237, 1981.

Murray, J. B.: Successful treatment of obsessive-compulsive disorders. *Genetic, Social, & General Psychology Monographs*, 112(2):173–199, 1986.

Mutter, C. B.: A hypno-therapeutic approach to exhibitionism: Outpatient therapeutic strategy. *Journal of Forensic Sciences*, 26(1):129–133, 1981.

Myall, R. W., Collins, F. J., Ross, A., et al.: Chronic factitious illness: Recognition and management of deception. *Journal of Oral and Maxillofacial Surgery*, 42(2):97–100, 1984.

Myers, E. D., & Calvert, E. J.: Information, compliance and side effects: A study of patients on antidepressant medication. *British Journal of Clinical Pharmacology*, 17(1):21–25, 1984.

Naylor, G. J., & Martin, B.: A double-blind out-patient trial of indalpine vs. mianserin. *British Journal of Psychiatry*, 147: 306–309, 1985.

Neborsky, R., Janowsky, D., Munson, E., et al.: Rapid treatment of acute psychotic symptoms with high- and low-dose haloperidol: Behavioral considerations. *Archives of General Psychiatry*, 38: 195–199, 1981.

Neidigh, L., & Kinder, B. N.: The use of audiovisual materials in sex therapy: A critical overview. *Journal of Sex & Marital Therapy*, 13(1):64–72, 1987.

Nemiah, J. C.: Dissociative disorders (hysterical neurosis, dissociative type). In H. I. Kaplan, A. M. Freedman, & B. J. Sadock (Eds.), *Comprehensive Textbook of Psychiatry*, 3rd ed., vol. 2. Baltimore, MD: Williams & Wilkins, 1980.

Nestoros, J. N., Suranyi-Cadotte, B. E., Spees, R. C., et al.: Diazepam in high doses is effective in schizophrenia. *Progress in Neuro-Psychopharmacology and Biological Psychiatry*, 6(4–6):513–516, 1982.

Newton, R. E., Marunycz, J. D., Alderdice, M. T., et al.: Review of the side-effect profile of buspirone. *American Journal of Medicine*, 80(3b):17–21, 1986.

Noyes, R., Jr., Chaudry, D. R., & Domingo, D. V.: Pharmacologic treatment of phobic disorders. *Journal of Clinical Psychiatry*, 47(9):445–452, 1986.

Nurnberg, H. G.: Survey of psychotherapeutic approaches to narcissistic personality disorder. *Hillside Journal of Clinical Psychiatry*, 6(2):204–220, 1984.

Nurnberg, H. G., & Feldman, A.: Hospital management of borderline patients. In J. H. Masserman (Ed.), *Current Psychiatric Therapies, Volume 22*. New York: Grune & Stratton, 1983, pp. 221–229.

Nurnberg, H. G., & Levine, P. E.: Schizophrenia and antipsychotic drugs. *Comprehensive Therapeutics*, 12(10):42–52, 1986.

O'Connell, R. A., Mayo, J. A., Eng, L. K., et al.: Social support and long-term lithium outcome. *British Journal of Psychiatry*, 147:272–275, 1985.

O'Regan, J. B.: Hypersomnia and MAOI antidepressants. *Canadian Medical Association Journal*, 111:213, 1974.

Orne, M. T.: The use and misuse of hypnosis in court. *International Journal of Clinical and Experimental Hypnosis*, 27(4):311–341, 1979.

Osborne, M., Crayton, J. W., Javaid, J., et al.: Lack of effect of a gluten-free diet on neuroleptic blood levels in schizophrenic patients. *Biological Psychiatry*, 17(5):627–629, 1982.

Oswald, I.: Symptoms that depress the doctor: Insomnia. *British Journal of Sleep Medicine*, 31:219–224, 1984.

Pare, C. M.: The present status of monoamine oxidase inhibitors. *British Journal of Psychiatry*, 146:576–584, 1985.

Parkes, J. D.: Daytime drowsiness. *Lancet*, 2:1213–1218, 1981.

Parsons, C. L.: Group reminiscence therapy and levels of depression in the elderly. *Nurse Practitioner*, 11(3):68–76, 1986.

Pathy, M. S. J., Bayer, A. J., & Stoker, M. J.: A double-blind comparison of chloramathiazole and temazepam in elderly patients with sleep disturbance. *Acta Psychiatrica Scandinavica*, 73(329):99–103, 1986.

Pecknold, J. C., & Fleury, D.: Alprazolam-induced manic episode in two patients with panic disorder. *American Journal of Psychiatry*, 143(5):652–653, 1986.

Perenyi, A., Szuchs, R., & Frecska, E.: Tardive dyskinesia in patients receiving lithium maintenance therapy. *Biological Psychiatry*, 19(11):1573–1578, 1984.

Perry, J. C., & Flannery, R. B.: Passive-aggressive personality disorder. Treatment implications of a clinical typology. *Journal of Nervous and Mental Disease*, 170(3):164–173, 1982.

Peteet, J. R., & Gutheil, T. G.: The hospital and the borderline patient: Management guidelines for the community mental health center. *Psychiatric Quarterly*, 51(2):106–118, 1979.

Petrie, W. M., Van, T. A., Berney, S., et al.: Loxapine in psychogeriatrics: A placebo and standard controlled clinical investigation. *Journal of Clinical Psychopharmacology*, 2:122–126, 1982.

Pickar, D., Wolkowitz, O. M., Doran, A. R., et al.: Clinical and biochemical effects of verapamil administration to schizophrenic patients. *Archives of General Psychiatry*, 44(2):113–118, 1987.

Pickard Bartanian, F., Bunney, W. E., Maier, H. P., et al.: Short-term naloxone administration in schizophrenic and traumatic patients: A world health organization collaborative study. *Archives of General Psychiatry*, 39:313–318, 1982.

Plakun, E. M., Burkhardt, T. E., & Muller, J. T.: Fourteen-year follow-up of borderline and schizotypal personality disorders. *Comprehensive Psychiatry*, 26(5):448–455, 1985.

Pollack, M. H., Tesar, G. E., Rosenbaum, J. F., et al.: Clonazepam in the treatment of panic disorder and agoraphobia: A one-year follow-up. *Journal of Clinical Psychopharmacology*, 6(5):302–304, 1986.

Potkin, S. G., Weinberger, D., Kleinman, J., et al.: Wheat gluten challenge in schizophrenic patients. *American Journal of Psychiatry*, 138(9):1208–1211, 1981.

Pottash, A. L. C., Gold, M. S., & Extein, I.: The use of the clinical laboratory. In L. I. Sederer (Ed.), *Inpatient Psychiatry: Diagnosis and Treatment* (2nd Edition). Baltimore: Williams & Wilkins, 1986, pp. 197–218.

Prasad, A.: Efficacy of trazodone as an anti-obsessional agent. *Neuropsychobiology*, 15(Supplement 1):19–21, 1986.

Preskorn, S. H., & Othmer, S. C.: Evaluation of buproprion hydrochloride: The first of a new class of atypical antidepressants. *Pharmacotherapy*, 4:20–34, 1984.

Price, W. A., & Giannini, A. J.: Neurotoxicity caused by lithium-verapamil synergism. *Journal of Clinical Pharmacology*, 26(8):717–719, 1986.

Prien, R. F., Kupfer, D. J., Mansky, P. A., et al.: Drug therapy and the prevention of recurrence in unipolar and bipolar affective disorders. Report of the NIMH collaborative study group comparing lithium carbonate, imipramine, and a lithium carbonate–imipramine combination. *Archives of General Psychiatry*, 41(11):1096–1104, 1984.

Puzynski, S., & Klosiewicz, L.: Valproic acid amide in the treatment of affective and schizoaffective disorders. *Journal of Affective Disorders*, 6(1):115–121, 1984.

Quality Assurance Project: Treatment outlines for the management of anxiety states. *Australia and New Zealand Journal of Psychiatry*, 19(2):138–151, 1985a.

Quality Assurance Project: Treatment outlines for the management of obsessive-compulsive disorders. *Australia and New Zealand Journal of Psychiatry*, 19(3):240–253, 1985b.

Rabiner, C. J., Wegner, J. T., & Kane, J. M.: Outcome study of first-episode psychosis. I: Relapse rates after one year. *American Journal of Psychiatry*, 143(9):1155–1158, 1986.

Ragheb, M.: Ibuprofen can increase serum lithium level in lithium-treated patients. *Journal of Clinical Psychiatry*, 48(4):161–163, 1987.

Rajagopal, K. R., Abbrecht, P. H., & Jabbari, B.: Effects of medroxyprogesterone acetate in obstructive sleep apnea. *Chest*, 90(6):815–821, 1986.

Ramirez, L. F., McCormick, R. A., Russo, A. M., et al.: Patterns of substance abuse in pathological gamblers undergoing treatment. *Addictive Behaviors*, 8(4):425–428, 1983.

Rampertaap, M. P.: Neuroleptic malignant syndrome. *Southern Medical Journal*, 79(3): 331–336, 1986.

Rankin, H.: Control rather than abstinence as a goal in the treatment of excessive gambling. *Behaviour Research and Therapy,* 20(2):185–187, 1982.

Rasmussen, S. A.: Lithium and tryptophan augmentation in clomipramine-resistant obsessive-compulsive disorder. *American Journal of Psychiatry,* 141(10):1283–1285, 1984.

Ratey, J. J., Sands, S., & O'Driscoll, G.: The phenomenology of recovery in the chronic schizophrenic. *Psychiatry,* 49(4):277–289, 1986.

Reich, J.: The relationship between antisocial behavior and affective illness. *Comprehensive Psychiatry,* 26(3):296–303, 1985.

Reich, P., & Gottfried, L. A.: Factitious disorders in a teaching hospital. *Annals of Internal Medicine,* 99(2):240–247, 1983.

Reid, W. H.: Treatment of somnambulism in military trainees. *American Journal of Psychotherapy,* 29(1):101–106, 1975.

Reid, W. H.: Antisocial personality and related syndromes. In J. R. Lion (Ed.), *Personality Disorders: Diagnosis and Management.* Baltimore: Williams & Wilkins, 1981a.

Reid, W. H. (Ed.):*The Treatment of Antisocial Syndromes.* New York: Van Nostrand Reinhold, 1981b.

Reid, W. H.: *Treatment of the DSM-III Psychiatric Disorders.* New York: Brunner/Mazel, 1983.

Reid, W. H.: The antisocial personality: A review. *Hospital and Community Psychiatry,* 36(8):831–837, 1985.

Reid, W. H.: Antisocial personality. In R. M. Michels & J. O. Cavenar, Jr. (Eds.), *Psychiatry.* Philadelphia: J. B. Lippincott, 1986.

Reid, W. H., Ahmed, I., & Levie, C. A.: Treatment of sleepwalking: A controlled study. *American Journal of Psychotherapy,* 35(1):27–37, 1981.

Reid, W. H., Blouin, P., & Schermer, M.: A review of psychotropic medications and the glaucomas. *International Pharmacopsychiatry,* 11(3):163–174, 1976.

Reid, W. H., & Gutnik, B. D.: Organic treatment of chronically violent patients. *Psychiatric Annals,* 12(5):526–542, 1982.

Reid, W. H., Haffke, E. A., & Chu, C. C.: Diazepam in treatment of intractable sleepwalking. *Hillside Journal of Clinical Psychiatry,* 6(1):49–55, 1984.

Reid, W. H., & Matthews, W.: A wilderness experience treatment program for antisocial offenders. *International Journal of Offender Therapy and Comparative Criminology,* 24(2):171–178, 1980.

Reid, W. H., & Solomon, G. H.: Community-based offender programs. In W. H. Reid (Ed.), *The Treatment of Antisocial Syndromes.* New York: Van Nostrand Reinhold, 1981.

Richardson, G. S., Carskadon, M. A., Flagg, W., et al.: Excessive daytime sleepiness in man: Multiple sleep latency measurement in narcoleptic and controlled subjects. *Electroencephalography & Clinical Neurophysiology,* 45:621–627, 1978.

Richelson, E.: Schizophrenia: Treatment. In R. Michaels & J. O. Cavenar, Jr., et al. (Eds.), *Psychiatry, Volume 1.* New York: J. B. Lippincott, 1986.

Rickels, K., Morris, R. J., Mauriello, R., et al.: Brotizolam, a triazolothiendodiazepine in insomnia. *Clinical Pharmacology and Therapy,* 40:293–299, 1986.

Ries, R. K., Bokan, J. A., Katon, W. J., et al.: The medical care abuser: Differential diagnosis and management. *Journal of Family Practice,* 13(2):257–265, 1981.

Rifkin, A., Quitkin, F., Carillo, C., et al.: Lithium treatment in emotionally unstable character disorders. *Archives of General Psychiatry,* 27:519–523, 1972.

Rifkin, A., & Siris, S. G.: Panic disorder: Response to sodium lactate and treatment with antidepressants. *Progress in Neuro-Psychopharmacology and Biological Psychiatry,* 9(1):33–38, 1985.

Rihmer, Z., Arato, M., Gyorgy, S., et al.: Dexamethasone suppression test as an aid for selection of specific antidepressant drugs in patient with endogenous depression. *Pharmacopsychiatry,* 18(5):306–308, 1985.

Ritzler, B. A.: Paranoia—Prognosis and treatment: A review. *Schizophrenia Bulletin,* 7(4) 710–728, 1981.

Robey, A.: Personal communication, 1981.

Robinson, A. D., & McCreadie, R. G.: The nithsdale schizophrenia survey. V. Follow-up of tardive dyskinesia at 3½ years. *British General Psychiatry*, 149:621–623, 1986.

Roselaar, S. E., Langdon, N., Lock, C. B., et al.: Selegiline in narcolepsy. *Sleep*, 10(5):491–495, 1987.

Rosenbaum, M. B.: Sex therapy today. *Bulletin of the Menninger Clinic*, 49(3):270–279, 1985.

Rosenbaum, M. S.: Treating hair-pulling in a seven-year-old male: Modified habit reversal for use in pediatric settings. *Journal of Development and Behavioral Pediatrics*, 3(4):241–242, 1982.

Rosenbluth, M.: The inpatient treatment of the borderline personality disorder: A critical review and discussion of aftercare implications. *Canadian Journal of Psychiatry*, 32(3):228–237, 1987.

Rosenthal, M. S.: Therapeutic communities: A treatment alternative for many but not all. *Journal of Substance Abuse Treatment*, 1(1):55–58, 1984.

Ross, W. P., Schultz, J. R., & Edelstein, P.: The biopsychosocial approach: Clinical examples from a consultation-liaison service. *Psychosomatics*, 23(2):141–151, 1982.

Roth, T., Zorick, F., Wittig, R., et al.: Pharmacological and medical considerations in hypnotic use. *Sleep*, 5:S46–S52, 1982.

Rowlands, D.: Therapeutic touch: Its effects on the depressed elderly. *Australian Nurses Journal*, 13(11):45–52, 1984.

Ruedrich, S. L., Chu, C. C., & Wadle, C. V.: The amytal interview in the treatment of psychogenic amnesia. *Hospital and Community Psychiatry*, 26(10):1045–1046, 1985.

Rush, A. J.: Diagnosis of affective disorders. In A. J. Rush & K. Z. Altshuler (Eds.), *Depression: Basic Mechanisms, Diagnosis, and Treatment*. New York: Guilford Press, 1986, pp. 1–31.

Rush, A. J., Beck, A. T., Kovacs, M., et al.: Comparative efficacy of cognitive therapy and pharmacotherapy in the treatment of depressed outpatients. *Cognitive Therapy and Research*, 1:17, 1977.

Rush, A. J., Beck, A. T., Kovacs, M., et al.: Comparison of the effects of cognitive therapy and pharmacotherapy on hopelessness and self-concept. *American Journal of Psychiatry*, 139:862–866, 1982.

Russo, A. M., Taber, J. I., McCormick, R. A., et al.: An outcome study of an inpatient treatment program for pathological gamblers. *Hospital and Community Psychiatry*, 35(8):823–827, 1984.

Sachs, C., Persson, H. E., & Hagenfeldt, K.: Menstruation-related periodic hypersomnia: A case study with successful treatment. *Neurology*, 32(12):1376–1379, 1982.

Salzman, C.: The use of ECT in the treatment schizophrenia. *American Journal of Psychiatry*, 137: 1032, 1980.

Salzman, C., Green, A. I., Rodriguez-Villa, F., et al.: Benzodiazepines combined with neuroleptics for acute and severe disruptive behavior. *Psychosomatics*, 27 (Supplement):17–21, 1987.

Salzman, L.: Psychotherapeutic management of obsessive-compulsive patients. *American Journal of Psychotherapy*, 39(3):323–330, 1985.

Saul, T., Jones, B. P., Edwards, K. G., et al.: Randomized comparison of atenolol and placebo in the treatment of anxiety: A double-blind study. *European Journal of Clinical Pharmacology*, 28(Supplement):109–110, 1985.

Scarzella, L., Scarzella, R., Mailland, F., et al.: Amineptine in the management of the depressive syndromes. *Progress in Neuro-Psychopharmacology and Biological Psychiatry*, 9(4):429–439, 1985.

Schmidt, K.: Pipothiazine palmitate: A versatile, sustained-action neuroleptic in the psychiatric practice. *Current Medical Research and Opinion* (England), 10(5):326–329, 1986.

Schneider-Helmert, D.: DSIP in sleep disturbances. *European Neurology*, 25(2):154–157, 1986.

Schneider-Helmert, D., & Spinweber, C. L.: Evaluation of L-tryptophan for treatment of insomnia: A review. *Psychopharmacology* (Berlin), 89:1–7, 1986.

Schnitt, J. M., & Nocks, J. J.: Alcoholism treatment of Vietnam veterans with post-traumatic stress disorder. *Journal of Substance Abuse Treatment*, 1(3):179–189, 1984.

Schover, L. R., & vonEschenbach, A. C.: Sex therapy and the penile prosthesis: A synthesis. *Journal of Sex & Marital Therapy*, 11(1):57–66, 1985.

Schover, L. R., vonEschenbach, A. C., Smith, D. B., et al.: Sexual rehabilitation of urologic cancer patients. A practical approach. *CA*, 34(2):66–74, 1984.

Schreter, R. K.: Treating the untreatable: A group experience with somaticizing borderline patients. *International Journal of Psychiatry and Medicine*, 10(3):205–215, 1980.

Schwartz, L. S., Robinson, M. V., Flaherty, J. A., et al.: A supportive care clinic: Maintaining the chronic psychiatric patient. *Hillside Journal of Clinical Psychiatry*, 8(2):202–208, 1986.

Sederer, L. I., & Thorbeck, J.: First do no harm: Short-term inpatient psychotherapy of the borderline patient. *Hospital and Community Psychiatry*, 37(7):692–697, 1986.

Seidel, W. F., Cohen, S. A., Bliwise, N. G., et al.: Dose-related effects of triazolam and flurazepam on a circadian rhythm insomnia. *Clinical Pharmacology and Therapeutics*, 40:31420, 1986.

Serban, G., & Siegel, S.: Response of borderline and schizotypal patients to small doses of thiothixene and haloperidol. *American Journal of Psychiatry*, 141(11):1455–1458, 1984.

Shah, J. H., DeLeon-Jones, F. A., Schickler, R., et al.: Symptomatic reactive hypoglycemia during glucose tolerance tests in lithium-treated patients. *Metabolism*, 35(7):634–639, 1986.

Shalev, A., & Munitz, H.: Conversion without hysteria: A case report and review of literature. *British Journal of Psychiatry*, 148:198–203, 1986.

Shapira, B., Oppenheim, G., Zohar, J., et al.: Lack of efficacy of estrogen supplementation to imipramine in resistant female depressives. *Biological Psychiatry*, 20(5):576–579, 1985.

Shapiro, W. R.: Treatment of cataplexy with clomipramine. *Archives of Neurology*, 32:653–656, 1975.

Sheline, Y. I., & Miller, M. B.: Catatonia relieved by oral diazepam in a patient with a pituitary microadenoma. *Psychosomatics*, 27(12):860–862, 1986.

Shively, D., & Petrich, J.: Correctional mental health. *Psychiatric Clinics of North America*, 8(3):537–550, 1985.

Shukla, S., Cook, B. L., & Miller, M. G.: Lithium-carbamazepine vs lithium-neuroleptic prophylaxis in bipolar illness. *Journal of Affective Disorders*, 9(3):219–222, 1985.

Siebel, M. M., Freeman, M. G., & Graves, W. L.: Carcinoma of the cervix and sexual functioning. *Obstetrics and Gynecology*, 55(4):484–487, 1980.

Sifneos, P. E.: Short-term dynamic psychotherapy for patients with physical symptomatology. *Psychotherapy and Psychosomatics*, 42(1–4):48–51, 1984.

Sifneos, P. E.: Short-term dynamic psychotherapy of phobic and mildly obsessive-compulsive patients. *American Journal of Psychotherapy*, 39(3):314–322, 1985.

Silver, D.: Psychotherapy of the characterologically difficult patient. *Canadian Journal of Psychiatry*, 28(7):513–521, 1983.

Silver, D.: Psychodynamics and psychotherapeutic management of the self-destructive character-disordered patient. *Psychiatric Clinics of North America*, 8(2):357–375, 1985.

Simmons, D. A., Daamen, M. J., Harrison, J. W., et al.: Hospital management of a patient with factitial dermatitis. *General Hospital Psychiatry*, 9(2):147–150, 1987.

Simon, J. I.: Day hospital treatment for borderline adolescents. *Adolescence*, 21(83):561–572, 1986.

Simons, A. D., Levine, J. L., Lustman, P. J., et al.: Patient attrition in a comparative outcome study of depression: A follow-up report. *Journal of Affective Disorders*, 6:163, 1984.

Simpson, G. M., Pi, E. H., & Sramek, J. J., Jr.: Neuroleptics and antipsychotics. In N. B. Blackwell (Ed.), Meyler's Side Effects of Drugs (Tenth Edition). New York: Elsevier, 1984.

Smith, P. L., Haponik, E. F., Allen, R. P., et al.: The effects of protriptylene in sleep-disordered breathing. American Review of Respiratory Diseases, 127(1):8–13, 1983.

Smith, P. L., Haponik, E. F., & Bleeker, E. R.: The effects of oxygen in patients with sleep apnea. American Review of Respiratory Diseases, 130:985–963, 1984.

Smith, R. C.: A clinical approach to the somatizing patient. Journal of Family Practice, 21(4):294–301, 1985.

Smith, R. C., Veroulis, G., Shvartsburd, A., et al.: RBC and plasma levels of haloperidol and clinical response in schizophrenia. American Journal of Psychiatry, 139:1054, 1982.

Snaith, R. P., & Collins, S. A.: Five exhibitionists and a method of treatment. British Journal of Psychiatry, 138: 126–130, 1981.

Snyder, D. K., & Berg, P.: Predicting couples' response to brief directive sex therapy. Journal of Sex & Marital Therapy, 9(2):114–120, 1983.

Snyder, S.: Trichotillomania treated with amitriptyline. Journal of Nervous and Mental Disease, 168(8):505–507, 1980.

Socarides, C. W.: Some problems encountered in psychoanalytic treatment of overt male homosexuality. American Journal of Psychotherapy, 33(4):506–520, 1979.

Soloff, P. H., George, A., Nathan, R. S., et al.: Progress in pharmacotherapy of borderline disorders. A double-blind study of amitriptyline, haloperidol, and placebo. Archives of General Psychiatry, 43(7):691–697, 1986a.

Soloff, P. H., George, A., Nathan, S., et al.: Amitriptyline and haloperidol in unstable and schizotypal borderline disorders. Psychopharmacology Bulletin, 22(1):177–182, 1986b.

Soloff, P. H., George, A., Nathan, R. S., et al.: Paradoxical effects of amitriptyline on borderline patients. American Journal of Psychiatry, 143(12):1603–1605, 1986c.

Solomon, L., & Williamson, P.: Verapamil in bipolar illness. Canadian Journal of Psychiatry, 31(5):442–444, 1986.

Spencer, J.: Maximization of biofeedback following cognitive stress preselection in generalized anxiety. Perceptual and Motor Skills, 63(1):239–242, 1986.

Spiegel, D.: Multiple personality of a post-traumatic stress disorder. Psychiatric Clinics of North America, 7(1):101–110, 1984.

Spielman, A. J., Saskin, P., & Thorpy, M. J.: Treatment of chronic insomnia by restriction of time in bed. Sleep, 10(1):45–56, 1987.

Spiker, B. G., Hanin, I., Cofsky, J., et al.: Pharmacological treatment of delusional depressives. Psychopharmacology Bulletin, 17:201–202, 1981.

Squire, L. R., & Slater, P. C.: Electroconvulsive therapy and complaints of memory dysfunction: A prospective three-year follow-up study. British Journal of Psychiatry, 142: 1, 1983.

Sranek, J. J., Simpson, G. N., Morrison, R. L., et al.: A prospective study of anticholinergic agents for prophylaxis of neuroleptic-induced dystonic reactions. Journal of Psychiatry, 47:305–309, 1986.

Stern, B. A., Fromm, M. G., & Sacksteder, J. L.: From coercion to collaboration: Two weeks in the life of a therapeutic community. Psychiatry, 49(1):18–32, 1986.

Stevens, M. J.: Behavioral treatment of trichotillomania. Psychological Reports, 55:987–990, 1984.

Stewart, J. W., Harrison, W., Quitkin, F., et al.: Phenelzine-induced pyridoxine deficiency. Journal of Clinical Psychopharmacology, 4:225–226, 1984.

Sticher, M., Abramovits, W., & Newcomer, V. V.: Trichotillomania in adults. Cutis, 26(1):90, 97–101, 1980.

Stone, J. L., McDaniel, K. D., Hughes, J. R., et al.: Episodic dyscontrol disorder and paroxysmal EEG abnormalities: Successful treatment with carbamazepine. Biological Psychiatry, 21(2):208–212, 1986.

Stone, M. H.: Schizotypal personality: Psychotherapeutic aspects. *Schizophrenia Bulletin,* 11(4):576–589, 1985a.

Stone, M. H.: Analytically oriented psychotherapy in schizotypal and borderline patients: At the border of treatability. *Yale Journal of Biological Medicine,* 58(3):275–288, 1985b.

Stone, M. H.: Borderline personality disorder. In R. Michels, J. O. Cavenar, Jr., et al. (Eds.), *Psychiatry, Volume I.* Philadelphia: J. B. Lippincott, 1986.

Stone, M. H.: Psychotherapy of borderline patients in light of long-term follow-up. *Bulletin of the Menninger Clinic,* 51(3):231–347, 1987.

Storms, L. H., Clopton, J. M., & Wright, C.: Effects of gluten on schizophrenics. *Archives of General Psychiatry,* 39(3):323–327, 1982.

Strain, J. J.: Diagnostic considerations in the medical setting. *Psychiatric Clinics of North America,* 4(2):287–300, 1981.

Strider, F. D., & Menolascino, F. J.: Treatment of antisocial syndromes in the mentally retarded. In W. H. Reid (Ed.), *The Treatment of Antisocial Syndromes.* New York: Van Nostrand Reinhold, 1981.

Stringer, A. Y., & Josef, N. C.: Methylphenidate in the treatment of aggression in two patients with antisocial personality disorder. *American Journal of Psychiatry,* 140(10):1365–1366, 1983.

Stromgren, L. S., & Boller, S.: Carbamazepine in treatment and prophylaxis of manic-depressive disorder. *Psychiat. Dev.,* 3(4):349–367, 1985.

Stürup, G. K., & Reid, W. H.: Herstedvester: An historical overview of institutional treatment. In W. H. Reid (Ed.), *The Treatment of Antisocial Syndromes.* New York: Van Nostrand Reinhold, 1981.

Szapocznik, J., Kurtines, W. M., Santisteban, D., et al.: Ethnic and cultural variations in the care of the aged. New directions in the treatment of depression in the elderly: A life enhancement counseling approach. *Journal of Geriatric Psychiatry,* 15(2):257–281, 1982.

Szasz, G., Paty, D., & Maurice, W. L.: Sexual dysfunctions in multiple sclerosis. *Annals of the New York Academy of Sciences,* 436:443–452, 1984.

Szymanski, H. V., Simon, J. C., & Gutterman, N.: Recovery from schizophrenic psychosis. *American Journal of Psychiatry,* 140(3):335–338, 1983.

Taber, J. I., McCormick, R. A., Russo, A. M., et al.: Follow-up of pathological gamblers after treatment. *American Journal of Psychiatry,* 144(6):757–761, 1987.

Takeda, M., Tanino, S., Nishinuma, K., et al.: A case of hypophyseal prolactinoma with treatable delusions of dermatozoiasis. *Acta Psychiatrica Scandinavica,* 72(5):470–475, 1985.

Talbott, J. A.: Chronic mental illness. *Audio Digest Psychiatry,* 11(2), January 1982.

Talley, J.: Geriatric depression: Avoiding the pitfalls of primary care. *Geriatrics,* 42(4):53–60, 65–66, 1987.

Tanney, B.: Electroconvulsive therapy and suicide. *Suicide and Life-Threatening Behavior,* 16(2):116–140, 1986.

Tarachow, S.: *An Introduction to Psychotherapy.* New York: International Universities Press, 1963.

Tarrier, N., & Main, C. J.: Applied relaxation training for generalised anxiety and panic attacks: The efficacy of a learnt coping strategy on subjective reports. *British Journal of Psychiatry,* 149:330–336, 1986.

Taylor, P., & Fleminger, J. J.: ECT for schizophrenia. *Lancet,* i: 1380, 1980.

Taylor, R. E.: Imagery for the treatment of obsessional behavior: A case study. *American Journal of Clinical Hypnosis,* 27(3):175–179, 1985.

Tearnan, B. H., Goetsch, V., & Adams, H. E.: Modification of disease phobia using a multi-faceted exposure program. *Journal of Behavior Therapy and Experimental Psychiatry,* 16(1):57–61, 1985.

Tesar, G. E., & Rosenbaum, J. F.: Successful use of clonazepam in patients with treatment-resistant panic disorder. *Journal of Nervous and Mental Disease,* 174(8):477–482, 1986.

Theorell, T.: Life events and manifestations of ischemic heart disease: Epidemiological and psychophysiological aspects. *Psychotherapy and Psychosomatics*, 34:135–148, 1980.

Thigpen, C. H., & Cleckley, H. M.: *The Three Faces of Eve.* New York: McGraw-Hill, 1957.

Thompson, C. J., & Baylis, P. H.: Asymptomatic Graves' disease during lithium therapy. *Postgraduate Medical Journal*, 62(726):295–296, 1986.

Thyer, B. A.: Audio-taped exposure therapy in the case of obsessional neurosis. *Journal of Behavioral Therapy and Experimental Psychiatry*, 16(3):271–273, 1985.

Tollefson, G.: Alprazolam in the treatment of obsessive symptoms. *Journal of Clinical Psychopharmacology*, 5(1):39–42, 1985.

Tolpin, T. H.: A change in the self: The development and transformation of an idealizing transference. *International Journal of Psychoanalysis*, 64(part 4):461–483, 1983.

Trabert, W., von Blohm, G., & Gawlitza, M.: Schwere Hypermatrianie Imrahmeneiner Katatomen Schizophrenie. *Forteschr. Neurol. Psychiatr.*, 54(6):196–198, 1986.

Tune, L. E., Creese, I., DePaulo, J. R., et al.: Clinical state and serum neuroleptic levels measured by radioreceptor assay in schizophrenia. *American Journal of Psychiatry*, 137: 187, 1980.

Tupin, J. P., Smith, D. B., Clannon, T. L., et al.: The long-term use of lithium in aggressive prisoners. *Comprehensive Psychiatry*, 13:209–214, 1972.

Vaamonde, C. A., Millian, N. E., Magrinat, G. S., et al.: Longitudinal evaluation of glomerular filtration rate during long-term lithium therapy. *American Journal of Kidney Diseases*, 7(3):213–216, 1986.

Van den Hoed, T., Kraemer, H., Guilleminault, C., et al.: Disorders of excessive daytime somnolence: Polygraphic and clinical data for 100 patients. *Sleep*, 4:23–37, 1981.

van Ree, J. M., Verhoeven, W. M., Claas, F. H., et al.: Antipsychotic action of gamma-type endorphins: Animal and human studies. *Progress in Brain Research*, 65: 221–235, 1986.

Varner, R. V., & Gaitz, C. M.: Schizophrenic and paranoid disorders in the aged. *Psychiatric Clinics of North America*, 5(1):107–118, 1982.

Vasile, R. G., Samson, J. A., Bemporad, J., et al.: A biopsychosocial approach to treating patients with affective disorders. *American Journal of Psychiatry*, 144(3):341–344, 1987.

Vestergaard, P., & Schou, M.: The effect of age on lithium dosage requirements. *Pharmacopsychiatry*, 17(6)199–201, 1984.

Vidalis, A. A., & Baker, G. H.: Factors influencing effectiveness of day hospital treatment. *International Journal of Social Psychiatry* (England), 32(3):3–8, 1986.

Videka-Sherman, L., & Lieberman, M.: The effects of self-help and psychotherapy intervention on child loss: The limits of recovery. *American Journal of Orthopsychiatry*, 55(1):70–82, 1985.

Viner, J.: Milieu concepts for short-term hospital treatment of borderline patients. *Psychiatric Quarterly*, 57(2):127–133, 1986.

Virkkunen, M.: Reactive hypoglycemic tendency among arsonists. *Acta Psychiatrica Scandinavica*, 69(5):445–452, 1984.

Vital-Herne, J., Gerbino, L., Kay, S. R., et al.: Mesoridazine and thioridazine: Clinical effects and blood levels in refractory schizophrenics. *Journal of Clinical Psychiatry*, 47(7):375–379, 1986.

Vlissides, D. N., Venulet, A., & Jenner, F. A.: A double-blind gluten-free/gluten-load controls trial in a secure ward population. *British Journal of Psychiatry*, 148:447–452, 1986.

Volavka, J., & Cooper, T. V.: Review of haloperidol blood level and clinical response: Looking through the window. *Journal of Clinical Psychopharmacology*, 7(1):25–30, 1987.